cut here

Pick of the Web: Essential Health and Fitness Sites

Make these sites your first stops for health and fitness information on the Web. Visit them all and bookmark your favorites so you can refer to them often.

Discovery Health   http://www.discoveryhealth.com

drkoop.com   http://www.drkoop.com

Fitness Partner Connection Jumpsite
http://www.primusweb.com/fitnesspartner

FitnessLink   http://www.fitnesslink.com

Hardin Meta Directory of Internet Health Sources
http://www.lib.uiowa.edu/hardin/md/index.html

HealthAtoZ   http://www.healthatoz.com

HealthCentral   http://www.healthcentral.com

HealthFinder   http://www.healthfinder.com

Intelihealth   http://www.intelihealth.com

Mayo Health Oasis   http://www.mayo.ivi.com

MEDLINEplus   http://www.nlm.nih.gov/medlineplus/

OnHealth   http://www.onhealth.com

Phys   http://www.phys.com

Quackwatch   http://www.quackwatch.com

ThriveOnline   http://www.thriveonline.com/

que®

The PILOT Method

How do you know whether you've found a credible Web site? The PILOT Method helps you evaluate it.

P Purpose

If the site has a mission statement, read it. If not, read the home page and analyze the site's purpose. Does it inform and educate? Or is it designed to persuade, sell, outrage, or entertain?

I Information

Truly useful Web sites offer valuable information and emphasize facts rather than opinion and testimonials. If the site is selling *anything*, ask yourself how that might influence the content.

L Links

The best sites want to inform you and are happy to recommend additional Web sites to further your knowledge in that topic or related topics. The best links are rated or reviewed.

O Originator

Who is responsible for the information? Best bets for sound health and fitness information are consumer-advocacy groups, health-professional organizations, well-known hospitals, and government- and university-sponsored sites.

T Timeliness

Depending on the topic you are looking into, the information should not be more than a few years old. Medical information should be more current. Look for sites that update frequently.

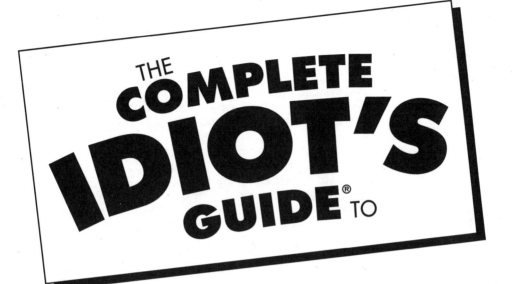

THE **COMPLETE IDIOT'S GUIDE®** TO

Online Health
and Fitness

Joan Price
Shannon Entin

alpha
books

A Division of Macmillan USA
201 W. 103rd Street, Indianapolis, IN 46290

Trademarks

Warning and Disclaimer

Associate Publisher
Greg Wiegand

Acquisitions Editor
Angelina Ward

Development Editor
Sarah Robbins

Managing Editor
Thomas F. Hayes

Project Editor
Tom Stevens

Copy Editor
Molly Schaller

Indexer
Sandra Henselmeier

Proofreader
Maribeth Echard

Technical Editor
Doug Dafforn

Illustrator
Judd Winick

Team Coordinator
Sharry Lee Gregory

Interior Designer
Nathan Clement

Cover Designer
Michael Freeland

Copy Writer
Eric Borgert

Production
Lisa England
Dan Harris
Brad Lenser

Contents at a Glance

Foreword   xiv

Introduction   1

Part 1: Finding Health and Fitness Information in
        Cyberspace   5

1 Why Use the Internet to Find Health and Fitness
  Information?   7
  *The power and pitfalls of using this rich information
  resource.*

2 What's Out There: The Many Faces of Online Health
  and Fitness Information   13
  *Learn to use search engines and Web directories and
  understand what you find.*

3 Junk or Jewel? Evaluating Web Site Content and
  Protecting Yourself   27
  *How to distinguish between reliable content, entertain-
  ment, and advertising when the lines are blurry.*

Part 2: Working Out on the Web   39

4 Developing Your Personal Fitness Program   41
  *Take your next—or first—steps in your personal shape-up
  plan.*

5 Aerobics: Raising Your Heart Rate Online   53
  *Online help to implement aerobic activities into your pro-
  gram.*

6 Strength Training: Not Just for Bodybuilders   65
  Time-tested basics for getting stronger.

7 Personal Trainers: Finding One That's Right for You   77
  *How to choose and use a personal trainer to help you
  reach your goals.*

8 Mind/Body Fitness: Stretching, Yoga, Martial Arts,
  and More   85
  *Enhance the quality of your workout program by includ-
  ing mind/body exercises.*

9 Recreational Activities: Fun and Fitness   93
  *Make exercise enjoyable with outdoor activities, dancing,
  and family fun.*

10 Fitness Shopping on the Web: Equipment and
   Accessories 103
   How to research what you need and buy it from a rep-
   utable source.

11 Hit the Road: Health and Fitness Resorts, Spas, and
   Vacations 113
   Take your fitness habit with you when you travel for busi-
   ness or pleasure.

Part 3: How to Find Nutrition, Diet, and Weight-Loss Information Online 121

12 Nutrition 101: Sorting It Out 123
   How to eat for health.

13 It's No Mystery: Losing Weight Safely and Effectively 135
   Find the facts and avoid the gimmicks.

14 Finding a Friend: Weight-Loss Support and Motivation
   Online 145
   Where to find online pep talks, pity parties, and motivat-
   ing friends for weight-loss support.

15 Promising the Moon: Beware of Fad Diets, Outrageous
   Claims, and Magic 153
   Sure-fire tips for recognizing the warning signs that a
   weight-loss plan will lighten only your wallet.

16 Accept It: Accepting Your Body and Your Weight 165
   Get off the diet roller coaster and live your life fully, what-
   ever your weight.

17 Cooking Up a Storm: Healthy Cooking Tips and Recipes
   Online 173
   Find healthy recipes and cooking tips online.

Part 4: How to Find and Evaluate Medical Resources Online 181

18 Under the Microscope: Researching Health Decisions
   and Evaluating Medical Web Sites 183
   Learn how to research a medical topic and assess what
   you find.

19 Alternative Medicine 195
   Explore different complementary therapies.

20 Kids' Health: Illnesses and Healthy Habits 205
   Find health information for and about children and
   teenagers.

21 Mental Health   215
Get help for mental illness, stress, and crises.

22 Check Before Swallowing: Medication   225
Learn about prescription drugs and herbs online.

**Part 5: Zeroing In: Researching Specific Medical
Conditions Online**   **237**

23 Menopause   239
Understand this life change and explore your options.

24 HIV/AIDS   247
Find the most credible and current HIV/AIDS information.

25 Cancer   255
Get cancer information and support online.

Glossary   **265**

Index   **269**

Contents

Introduction   **1**

How to Use This Book 1
Extras 2
Special Thanks 4

Part 1 Finding Health and Fitness Information in Cyberspace   **5**

1 Why Use the Internet to Find Health and Fitness Information?   **7**

Health and Fitness Through Your Computer? Yes! 8
   Information Available at the Click of a Mouse 8
   Depth and Breadth 8
An Invaluable Tool for Improving Quality of Life 9
   Education 9
   Research 10
   Support 11

2 What's Out There: The Many Faces of Online Health and Fitness Information   **13**

The Little Engine That Can: Intro to Search Engines 13
   Robots and Spiders and Crawlers, Oh My! 15
   Web Directories 16
   Metasearch Sites 17
Types of Web Sites 19
   Jump Sites: Links Galore! 19
   News and Information 19
   Magazines and Trade Publications 21
   FAQs 21
   Associations and Institutions 21
   Personal Pages 22
   Storefront Sites: Sell, Sell, Sell 22

CyberFriends: Mailing Lists, Newsgroups, Bulletin
    Boards, and Chat 22
    Finding and Using Mailing Lists 22
    Finding and Using Newsgroups 24
    Finding and Using Bulletin Boards 24
    Finding and Using Chat Rooms 25

**3 Junk or Jewel? Evaluating Web Site Content
     and Protecting Yourself   27**

Protect Yourself from Scams 28
    They Want Your Money! 28
    If It Sounds Too Good to Be True, It Probably Is 29
Evaluating Web Site Content: The PILOT Method 30
    Purpose 31
    Information 32
    Links 33
    Originator 34
    Timeliness 35
Start Here 36
Evaluation Grad School 37

Part 2 Working Out on the Web   39

4 Developing Your Personal Fitness Program   41

How Fit Are You? 41
    Determining Your Fitness Level 42
    Fitness Testing Information Online 42
Setting Reachable Goals 44
Developing Your Fitness Program 45
    *Use the Three Components of Fitness: Aerobics, Strength
     Training, and Stretching* 46
    Create a Realistic Plan and Stick to It! 47
Joining a Health Club Versus Working Out at Home 47
Using Software to Track Your Progress 49
    Online Tools to Help You Succeed 50
Finding Workout Programs Online: Advantages and
    Disadvantages 51
Start Here: Sites to Help You Develop Your Fitness
    Program 51

vii

5 Aerobics: Raising Your Heart Rate Online   53

What Is Aerobic Activity? 53
Why Do You Need Aerobic Activity? 54
   Cardiovascular Health 54
   Weight Loss/Control..55
   Stress Reduction: Exercise Makes You Feel Good!..................55
How Often, How Long, How Hard? 56
Put Away That Magazine! Understanding Intensity............57
Types of Aerobic Activity: Finding Info Online 59
   Walking..59
   Inline Skating..59
   Running 60
   Tennis/Squash 60
   Swimming 61
   Cycling 61
   Cardiovascular Machines 62
   Aerobic Exercise Classes/Videos 62
It Doesn't Have to Feel Like "Exercise" 64

6 Strength Training: Not Just for Bodybuilders   65

Important Reasons Why You Need to Strength Train 65
Understanding Strength-Training Basics............................67
   Reps and Sets 68
   How Much Weight? 68
   How Often? 68
Getting the Results You Want 70
Start Here: Basic Strength-Training Sites 70
Bodybuilding 73
Start Here: Bodybuilding Sites..73

7 Personal Trainers: Finding One That's Right for You   77

What Does a Trainer Do? 78
Do You Need a Trainer? The Pros and Cons.....................78
What to Look For: Finding a Trainer Online and Off 79
   Education 79
   Certification...79
   Experience 80
   Individualization 80

Professionalism 80
Policies 80
Liability Insurance 80
Fees 80
Personality 81
Personal Training via Email: Serious Scam Potential 82
Start Here: Searching for Personal Trainers Online.............84

8 Mind/Body Fitness: Stretching, Yoga, Martial Arts, and More　　85

Adding Awareness to Your Workout: The Mind/Body
　Connection 85
Mind/Body Exercise for a Fit, Healthy Body.......................86
Using the Web to Make the Connection 87
Stretching...87
Pilates 90
Martial Arts 91
Sports Psychology 92

9 Recreational Activities: Fun and Fitness　　93

Using the Web to Plan Outdoor Fitness Activities 93
Locating Clubs and Organizations Online 95
Get Up and Dance 97
But Is It Exercise?...97
Social Dancing..98
Dance Classes 98
Fitness with the Family 100

10 Fitness Shopping on the Web: Equipment and Accessories　　103

What Type of Equipment Do You Need? 103
Finding Fitness Products Online 106
Start Here: Equipment for Sale 106
Exercise Videos..108
Monitors and Calipers 109
Shopping Online—Is It Safe? 110
Count to Ten (or 100) Before Purchasing the
　Latest "Gadget" 111

11 Hit the Road: Health and Fitness Resorts, Spas, and Vacations **113**

Treat Yourself to a Healthy Vacation! 113
Taking Your Fitness Habit with You *114*
Become an Active Vacationer *115*
Finding a Resort or Spa on the Web 117
Traveling for Business or Pleasure: Finding a Hotel
with a Gym 118

Part 3 How to Find Nutrition, Diet, and Weight-Loss Information Online **121**

12 Nutrition 101: Sorting It Out **123**

You Are What You Eat 123
Calories *123*
Carbohydrates *125*
Proteins *126*
Fats *126*
Vitamins and Minerals *128*
What Exactly Is a "Healthy Diet"? 129
Online Advice Abounds 131
Start Here 132

13 It's No Mystery: Losing Weight Safely and Effectively **135**

The Business of Weight Loss 135
Calories In, Calories Out 136
Junk Food: Eat It, Wear It 137
Move It or You Won't Lose It 138
Unrealistic Expectations 139
Researching Weight Loss Online...140
Evaluating Weight-Loss Web Sites by Using the
PILOT Method 141
Sticking to It: Sites to Keep You Losing 142

14 Finding a Friend: Weight-Loss Support and Motivation Online   145

Commercial Support Groups.................................145
Online Support and Motivation 147
Mailing Lists 147
Newsgroups 147
Chat Rooms 148
Bulletin Boards 148
Email Pen Pals...150

15 Promising the Moon: Beware of Fad Diets, Outrageous Claims, and Magic   153

Why Diet Is a Four-Letter Word 153
What Do You Have to Lose? 154
Recognizing Quacky Diets and Weight-Loss Schemes 154
Spotting the Scams 155
Two Guys with a Placebo 156
Diet Books 158
Read Before You Buy: Reviews, Excerpts Online...............159
The Truth About Best-Selling Diet Books 159
Weight-Loss Red Flags 160
"Burns Fat" 161
"Gets Rid of Cellulite" 161
"Without Diet or Exercise" 162
Bozo Buzzwords: Magic, Secret, Easy, Effortless, Fast, Guaranteed, and Permanent...............................162
Scam Test 163

16 Accept It: Accepting Your Body and Your Weight   165

You Can Change Your Diet, but Not Your Genes.............165
How to Tell Whether You're Genetically Heavy...............166
What You Can or Can't Do About It 167
Self-Acceptance: Start Here 169

17 Cooking Up a Storm: Healthy Cooking Tips and Recipes Online **173**

Ingredients for Healthy Cooking 173
The Healthy Refrigerator 174
The Fresher, the Better 174
Great Substitutions...174
Expanding Your Mealtime Repertoire Using the Web 176
Learning More About Food 177
Learning More About Shopping..177
Cooking for Special Interests...178
Start Here: Recipe SuperSites 180

Part 4 How to Find and Evaluate Medical Resources Online **181**

18 Under the Microscope: Researching Health Decisions, Evaluating Medical Web Sites **183**

Personal Exam: What Are You Looking For? 184
How to Find—And Understand—Medical Journals 186
Medical Libraries 187
Buy Me: Products for Sale 188
PILOT Through the Internet 189
Purpose: Why Are They Offering You This? 189
Information: Content Considerations 190
Links: Do They Share You with Other Sites? 190
Originator: Who's in Charge?...190
Timeliness: Is It Current? 191
Start Here: Super Health/Medical Meta Sites 193

19 Alternative Medicine **195**

What Can You Find? 195
Acupuncture...197
Ayurvedic Medicine 197
Chinese Medicine 197
Chiropractic 197
Feldenkrais..198

Macrobiotics 198
Massage..198
Where's the Science? Fact Versus Fantasy, Opinion,
and Anecdote 199
I Believe: The Placebo Effect 200
Recognizing Red Flags 201
Start Here: Best Alternative/Complementary Sites 202

20 Kids' Health: Illnesses and Healthy Habits   205

Kids' Health for Parents....................................205
Researching Your Child's Illness Online 206
Parents Helping Parents 207
Kids' Health for Kids 209
Start Here: Healthy Kids' Web Sites....................210

21 Mental Health   215

Mental Health/Illness Resources 215
Crisis Help 216
Exploring Treatments and Therapies 218
The Virtual Couch: Online Therapists 218
You've Got a Friend: Support Groups Online...........220
Start Here: Best Mental Health Sites 221

22 Check Before Swallowing: Medication   225

Rx: What Can You Learn? 226
Buying Drugs Online..227
Online Pharmacies 227
No Prescription, No Drug 229
Herbal Medicine 229
Herbal Mix Alert 230
Herbs Online 230
Start Here: Drug Information Sites 234

Part 5 Zeroing In: Researching Specific Medical Conditions Online **237**

23 Menopause **239**

"They're Not Hot Flashes—They're Power Surges!": Symptoms 239
Treatment...240
   Conventional *241*
   Alternative *241*
Support...243
Start Here: Menopause Information Sites 243
Get Linked: More Than You Ever Thought You'd Find 245

24 HIV/AIDS **247**

Prevention 247
Testing 249
Treatment...249
Run, Don't Walk: Spotting Quacks 251
Research 251
Start Here: HIV/AIDS Info Sites 253

25 Cancer **255**

What Can You Find? 255
   Treatment Options *257*
   Support *258*
How to Research the Medical Literature...........................260
Start Here: Cancer Info and Support.................................261

Glossary **265**

Index **269**

Foreword

I've always encouraged my listeners and readers to seek out the best health information and advice available because there's a lot of bogus stuff floating around, especially on the Internet. The online revolution has made it easier to get good, solid information, but also to be bombarded by fraud and medical illiteracy.

This is an era of unprecedented medical progress and health education, and the Internet is playing a big and expanding role. I'm racing as hard as I can to keep my audience informed about what's fact, what's plausible, what's doubtful, and what's totally ridiculous. I'm happy to have the help of Joan Price and Shannon Entin in a book that teaches consumers how to find and evaluate online health, fitness, nutrition, and medical information.

I'm delighted by how friendly and easy to understand Joan and Shannon have made tough concepts, and how well they know both health and the Internet. This should be in the library of any newcomer to finding health information online—and even experienced readers will learn some new tricks.

—Dean Edell, M.D., media medical reporter and author of *Eat, Drink & Be Merry* (HarperCollins, 1999)

    http://healthcentral.com

Tell Us What You Think!

As the reader of this book, *you* are our most important critic and commentator. We value your opinion and want to know what we're doing right, what we could do better, what areas you'd like to see us publish in, and any other words of wisdom you're willing to pass our way.

As an Associate Publisher for Alpha Books, I welcome your comments. You can fax, email, or write me directly to let me know what you did or didn't like about this book—as well as what we can do to make our books stronger.

Please note that I cannot help you with technical problems related to the topic of this book, and that due to the high volume of mail I receive, I might not be able to reply to every message.

When you write, please be sure to include this book's title and author as well as your name and phone or fax number. I will carefully review your comments and share them with the author and editors who worked on the book.

Fax: 317-581-4666

Email: consumer@mcp.com

Mail: Greg Wiegand, Associate Publisher
           Alpha Books
           201 West 103rd Street

Introduction

Have you surfed the Net recently for health or fitness information? If you have, no doubt you found the sheer quantity of information overwhelming and intimidating, and you might have feared it would be impossible to master. You can't read everything—how can you possibly find the most useful information and know what to believe?

Ahem! That's our job. Whether you're a newbie (that's newcomer, in Netspeak) or an experienced surfer, our book aims to guide you and give you the tools for hacking your way through the jungle of online health information.

We point you to outstanding Web sites covering all aspects of health and fitness. More important, we teach you how to take control and find and evaluate sites yourself. As current as our information is as we get to press, we can't control whether a favorite Web site that we mention will disappear or change its URL (Web address), or if a better one will appear a month later. So, we see our job as empowering you to take charge. Part of that is teaching you how to steer away from scams, frauds, and misleading claims and advice, and toward respected, credible resources—and teaching you how to tell the difference.

How to Use This Book

Of course, we hope you'll read every word of this book (maybe two or three times!), but in all honesty, you don't have to read every chapter or go in order. We've organized this book into five parts. We recommend reading all of Part 1 first, because it has general information that applies, no matter what kind of health information you're seeking. Even if you skip around in Part 1, give your undivided attention to Chapter 3, "Junk or Jewel? Evaluating Web Site Content and Protecting Yourself"— the one absolutely essential chapter.

Part 1, "Finding Health and Fitness Information in Cyberspace," is an overview of how to locate online health resources and how to evaluate health sites on the World Wide Web.

Part 2, "Working Out on the Web," shows you how to get active and fit using the Internet to help you develop a program; find information about aerobics, strength training, recreational activities, and personal trainers; shop for fitness products; and keep up your fitness habit while traveling.

Part 3, "How to Find Nutrition, Diet, and Weight-Loss Information Online," introduces the basics of nutrition and healthy cooking, and tells you the truth about weight loss and diets.

Part 4, "How to Find and Evaluate Medical Resources Online," gives you a quick course in locating medical information, with a special emphasis on evaluating whether a Web site is credible. Chapters focus on alternative medicine, kids' health, mental health, and medications.

Part 5, "Zeroing In: Researching Specific Medical Conditions Online," shows you how to delve into a particular disease or condition. We explore menopause, HIV/AIDS, and cancer, pointing you to some superb sites and giving you tools for finding more.

Extras

You'll see these tips, cautions, and activities in boxes splashed throughout the book:

Get Up!

Quick fitness breaks and stretching activities that you can do while waiting for Web pages to load or search engines to search.

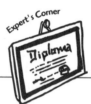

The Expert's Corner has quotes from experts in different health fields offering tips, comments, and cautions about getting accurate information.

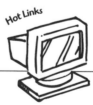

Hot Links

Unique Web sites that are worth a visit.

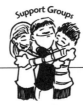

Support Groups

Newsgroups, mailing lists, chat, and bulletin boards to help you find the online support you need.

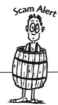

Scam Alert!

Warnings for avoiding frauds, rip-offs, and misleading advice.

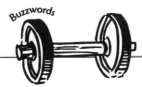

Buzzwords: Definitions of health, fitness, and Web terms.

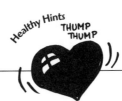

Healthy Hints

Tidbits of practical health information.

Special Thanks

Joan wants to thank her special friends—especially Joshua Boneh, Dan Goldes, John Martin, and Chris Overholt—who were so understanding when she scheduled working on this book ahead of all other plans and who listened when she talked of little else. She thanks her clients—especially Carol Augustine, Carolyn Goodwin, and Pat Lee—for their patience and flexibility at having their appointment times disrupted as deadlines approached. Thanks to Dan Goldes and Paul Roberts for reviewing the chapters in their areas of expertise. And many thanks to Chris Hendel for his invaluable research assistance.

Shannon would like to thank her husband Paul for his never-ending encouragement, for getting up at 5:30 a.m. with their son Logan while she banged away at the computer, and for being an incessant source of ideas and inspiration. She'd also like to thank her family—Alexandra, Janelle, Dick, Jane, Eileen, Joel, Jeff, Bev, Jared, and Kyle—for their love and understanding when she couldn't make family gatherings because of "the book."

Joan and Shannon thank each other for a collaboration made in cyber-heaven. Both owe special thanks to the whole team at Macmillan, especially Angelina Ward, acquisitions editor; to the medical experts who contributed their wisdom; and to all the people who generously provided content to the Web sites mentioned so that we can all be richer in knowledge.

Part 1

Finding Health and Fitness Information in Cyberspace

How many times have you bought the latest health or fitness book, only to find that the information was outdated—even outright wrong? Or, maybe you've listened to the diet guru of the moment on a TV talk show and wondered whether this information was valid and how you could check it out. The Internet is your ticket to valuable, in-depth, and timely information in the privacy of your home and with the ease of a mouse click. But where do you start? And how do you sift the quality information from the abundance of quackery and foolishness online?

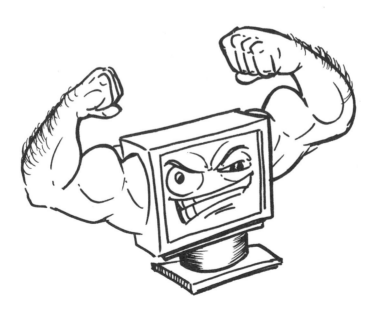

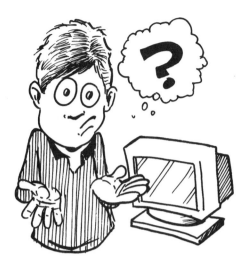

Chapter 1

Why Use the Internet to Find Health and Fitness Information?

In This Chapter

➤ Using the Internet to learn more about health and fitness topics

➤ Understanding the benefits and pitfalls of having vast amounts of information easily available online

Millions of Web sites are devoted to some aspect of health. It's impossible to pin down the number more precisely than that, because new sites go up and old sites go down faster than you can read this chapter. Also, defining a "health" site would take us longer than creating one. The medical, nutrition, weight loss, and fitness sites clearly qualify, but what about Aunt Agatha's magic cure for toothaches, or emu oil for skin cancer, arthritis, varicose veins, gangrene, Alzheimer's disease, and high cholesterol? You think we're making up that last one? It was an actual commercial site until the FDA barred it from making these medical claims recently.

The Internet—that vast network of unregulated data—has made health and fitness information more readily available now than it has been at any other time in history. This is a blessing as well as a curse. Although you can find answers to nearly any health or fitness question on the Internet, you might also find a mother lode of quacky sites and fraudulent products. This book is here to show you how to use the Internet at its best—as an invaluable tool for education, research, and support in your quest for a healthier lifestyle.

Health and Fitness Through Your Computer? Yes!

It sounds unlikely. How can sitting at your computer help you become healthier and fitter? The same way reading a manual can help you keep your car engine in tip-top shape. The special combination is education and action. Learn what steps to take for preventative maintenance of your body, adopt those steps, and your body will run like a well-oiled machine for many years to come.

If you have a disease or other medical condition, you can assist your doctor by visiting reputable sites and learning about symptoms, treatments, medications, the latest studies, and much more. Twenty-nine percent of Americans get medical information from the Internet—and 70 percent of these search online before visiting a doctor. One quarter of those who use the Internet to research medical information join online support groups. Using the Internet, you can find more information than you'd ever get from a single book—or even a library of books! And the information is available day or night, seven days a week.

The Internet is composed of three main tools you can use to further your education: email, newsgroups, and the popular World Wide Web. Each of these tools has its benefits and its pitfalls.

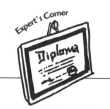

Expert's Corner

Diploma

"The best prescription is knowledge."

—Dr. C. Everett Koop, M.D., former U.S. Surgeon General and co-founder of http://www.drkoop.com

Information Available at the Click of a Mouse

According to a 1999 Harris poll, 60 million people searched the World Wide Web for health-care information in 1998—that's 68 percent of the 88 million people estimated to be online. Why such a large percentage? Simply put, the Internet provides boundless amounts of data at the click of a mouse.

Having all this data available has also complicated matters, because the information is largely unfiltered. Anyone can put up a Web page or pose as an "expert" in the anonymous world of the Internet.

In addition to searching for information online, you also need to evaluate its quality and reliability. Discussing health information found on the Internet with your doctor is always a good idea.

Depth and Breadth

"Take charge of your health!" we're told by healthcare plan providers, employers, and even our doctors. We are encouraged to learn more about how to eat better, get more active, quit smoking, prevent disease, and manage the health conditions we already have or are likely to get. Whew. As HMOs become the norm and the family doctor who makes house calls becomes a relic from the past, the burden of educating ourselves about health issues falls squarely on our shoulders.

The depth and breadth of information found on the Internet are astounding. When you search for a topic, you are likely to find thousands (often hundreds of thousands, sometimes millions!) of resources at your fingertips. Unlike going to a library and searching through a few books on a specific topic, the Web gives you instant access to virtually any topic and then links you to even more resources.

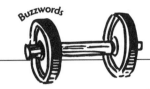

Buzzwords

Link: Short for hyperlink ; a reference to another document on the World Wide Web. Links are highlighted lines of text that take you to a Web site when you click them with your mouse.

An Invaluable Tool for Improving Quality of Life

What is your current state of health? Do you want to lose weight? Do you want to get in shape and have a healthier heart? Are you looking for answers about a medical condition? Are you in need of support in your quest for a healthier lifestyle?

Get Up

Stand and Deliver

Stand up! As ergonomic as your chair might be, get out of it at least every hour. Take "standing breaks" while you wait for a Web page, or, even better, pace the room quickly. Even just standing in place burns 25 percent more calories than sitting down. Pacing burns almost four times as many calories as sitting. Physical activity makes you feel less tired and helps your brain work better!

No matter where you are on the spectrum of health and fitness, the Internet can be your guide to a better quality of life.

Education

Education is your ticket to a long, happy, healthy life. Take the time to learn which foods you should be eating more and which you should be eating less, how much exercise is ideal for you, and how to reduce your stress levels and guard against illnesses.

Begin your education with a "meta site"—a Web site that offers tons of links and information on a broad range of topics. From there, you can link to more specific sites that focus on your area of interest. The following are two meta sites we like; HealthAtoZ is shown in Figure 1.1:

➤ The Fitness Partner Connection Jumpsite, http://www.primusWeb.com/fitnesspartner

➤ HealthAtoZ, http://www.healthatoz.com

Figure 1.1

HealthAtoZ is a top-notch site that provides its visitors with a broad range of health information.

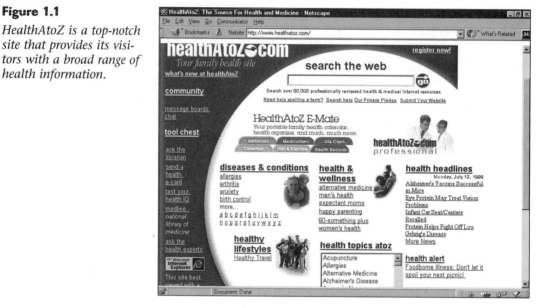

Research

If you're looking for in-depth, accurate, up-to-date information, you might want to bypass the many sites that claim to interpret health and medical findings, and go straight to the scientific sources. The World Wide Web tears down barriers and lets you access the same information that your doctor, nutritionist, or personal trainer reads (or should read!). Nowhere else can you find such a vast amount of information—and find it easily, after you learn a few skills. Many Web sites allow you to search through medical journals, databases of disease-related information, nutrition and food information, and more.

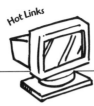

Hot Links

Mediconsult.com

`http://www.mediconsult.com`

This self-proclaimed "Virtual Medical Center" has it all—journal articles, educational materials, bulletin board support groups, current news, and drug information for a huge list of health/medical concerns.

Support

If you think the Internet is impersonal—think again. Whereas some people find true love in a chat room, you might find the support, motivation, and answers you need to achieve your fitness goals or cope with a disease or illness. Some sites are friendly and down to earth, such as Dean Edell's Health Central at `http://www.healthcentral.com`. And even when the best sources of information for a certain topic do more brain-filling than handholding, support groups help you personalize the information.

Get Up

Modem Push-Ups

While your modem is dialing and logging on, do push-ups against the desk. Place your hands about shoulder-width apart on the desk. Walk your feet away until your body makes a diagonal line from desk to floor. Keeping your back neutral (that is, not bent either forward or back), your abdominals tight, your chest high, and your shoulders down, bend your elbows, lowering your chest toward the desk. Exhale, straightening your elbows (do not lock them) and pushing yourself away from the desk. Repeat until your email is ready to read. Advanced: Do one-armed push-ups. Change arms each five repetitions. This exercise strengthens the chest, arms and shoulders, and makes the time pass.

The Least You Need to Know

➤ Although the information is unfiltered and must be evaluated for credibility, the Internet offers an astounding number of health and fitness resources.

➤ If you're looking to improve your quality of life by becoming healthier and fitter, the Internet can be used for education, research, and support.

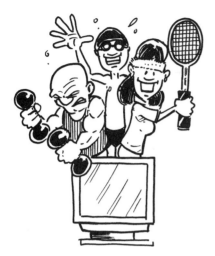

Chapter 2

What's Out There: The Many Faces of Online Health and Fitness Information

> ## In This Chapter
>
> ➤ Learning where to find information on the Internet
>
> ➤ Choosing and using search engines and Web directories effectively
>
> ➤ Understanding the different types of informational Web sites
>
> ➤ Using mailing lists, newsgroups, bulletin boards, and chat for friendship and support

You know the information you want is out there…somewhere. How do you find the Web site you want out of the tens (or hundreds!) of thousands on your topic? This chapter shows you how to be the train (chugging ahead with determination and direction) rather than the track (getting flattened and left behind) when you use search engines. We put you in the director's chair using Web directories.

The Little Engine That Can: Intro to Search Engines

Everyone who uses the World Wide Web has used a search engine—a Web site that enables you to search millions of Web pages for a given word or phrase. It's the most common way to locate info on the Web. You choose a search engine, key in a few words, and wait for results to flood your screen.

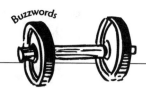

Buzzwords

Search Engine: A Web site that takes a word or phrase that you've typed and searches the Web for sites that relate to your query.

Get Up

Search Engine Locomotion

Get up and dance while you're waiting for the search engine to deliver the goods. Put on some motivating music (train theme is optional) and boogie, hip-hop, or tush-push your way around the room.

But search engines are not always the best way to find the information you want. Many people incorrectly assume that when they use a search tool, they are searching the "entire Web." This is far from true. The Web contains about 800 million pages (but who's counting?), and no one search engine catalogues more than 16 percent of the sites available to the public, according to a recent NEC Research Institute study reported in the journal *Nature* (July 8, 1999).

To make our search for information harder, the search engines are more likely to index commercial than educational and scientific sites. Try a search on "fitness" and you'll come up with hundreds of thousands of sites—some selling fitness products (or gimmicks!), some offering fitness advice, some promoting bodybuilders or models, and some with quality fitness information. But perhaps none of the sites that come up in your search result really answers your question. It takes some time—and knowledge of a few secrets—to pinpoint exactly what you're looking for on the Web.

The term "search engine" is often used to describe any type of search tool on the Internet. However, there are two distinct types of search tools: true search engines and Web directories. The difference between them is the way in which they compile their information. Your searching success depends on how well you use both of these tools.

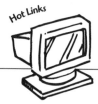

Hot Links

Search Engine Showdown

http://www.notess.com/search

The Search Engine Showdown is a great place to learn more about search engines. It offers a chart comparing search capabilities, reviews that tell you the engine's strengths and weaknesses, and tips to make the most of your search. This site covers not only traditional search engines, but also "meta" searches, newsgroup searches, and mailing list searches. Read about strategies to help you search the Web effectively, and find links to even more tools.

Robots and Spiders and Crawlers, Oh My!

True search engines utilize a type of software known as a "spider" (also called a "robot" or a "crawler"). The spider visits a Web site and "crawls" around its pages, forming an index of the site's content—essentially copying the site and saving it in its database. When you do a search by keying in a word, the search engine searches through the database of millions of Web pages that were copied by the spider to find that word, and it returns matching results to you.

Search engines are most useful if your search is simple, specific, and straightforward, and you want to find a comprehensive listing of what's available on the Web on this topic.

For example, let's say you want to find out about an asthma medication your physician has recommended, so you search "asthma inhaler." Use one search engine, and you might get 47,000 sites (we told you the Internet was vast!). So, narrow down your search as much as you can. Instead of "asthma inhaler," for example, search the name of the drug, such as Serevent. Ah, only 400 hits this time. (That still seems like a lot, but compared to 47,000, it's not so bad.)

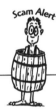

Scam Alert

Search Engines Do Not Evaluate Content!

A Web site that gets top billing from a search tool is automatically credible, right? Wrong! Some sites pay for top listings in search engines. Some use fancy programming tactics so that their page comes up even in a completely unrelated search. So, avoid the temptation to look just at the first sites at the head of the list of your search results—they might not be the best. You might, in fact, find something completely unrelated in the first few sites—grrrr.

Search engines are also helpful when you are looking for a unique topic. It's easier to find a needle in a haystack if the needle is something out of the ordinary, such as Joan's workout video, "The New LI Teknique," or very specific, such as "treadmill reviews."

If your search is general, broad, vague, or common, such as "exercise" or even "exercise videos," a directory is a better place to start. Some of the major search engines include HotBot (`http://www.hotbot.com`), Excite (`http://www.excite.com`), and AltaVista (`http://www.altavista.com`).

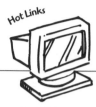

Searching the World Wide Web

```
http://www.lib.berkeley.edu/TeachingLib/Guides/Internet/
Strategies.html.
```

The University of California, Berkeley offers an excellent guide to analyzing your topic, choosing search tools, and using search strategies.

Web Directories

If you expect your search to result in a huge heap of information, or you want to spend an evening browsing through all sorts of related topics, a Web directory is the place to begin.

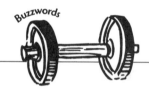

Browse: Like browsing the aisles in the grocery store, browsing the Web refers to visiting one Web site after another, looking for information that might interest you.

Web directories are compiled by human hand, unlike the "spiders" that search engines use to copy Web pages and compile indexes. Because sites are hand-picked and categorized into directory topics, you've got a better chance of finding something relevant when searching for a broad topic. A search engine matches your search term to any page containing that word; a Web directory finds sites that are chosen by a human being to match your request.

When you search using a directory site, such as Yahoo! (http://www.yahoo.com), Looksmart (http://www.looksmart.com) (see Figure 2.1), or Snap (http://www.snap.com), first try clicking on one of the categories on the home page, such as health. You should find a relevant list of sites you can visit to begin your research, whether you're looking for kickboxing or measles. If you don't find a category that matches your request, simply type in your search term and the directory guides you to related sites.

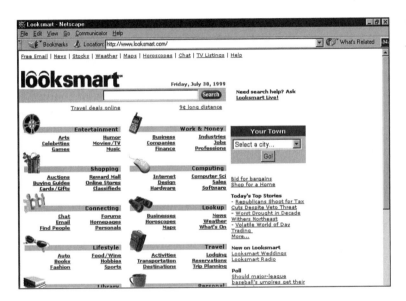

Figure 2.1

Looksmart.com offers news, weather, horoscopes, stocks, maps, and even TV listings in addition to its Web directory search tool.

Metasearch Sites

If you're looking for a "quick-and-dirty" overview of what's on the Web on a given topic, try a metasearch site. These sites submit your request to several search engines at the same time and return the integrated results to you. Advantage: It's faster than visiting one search page after another and typing in your request. Disadvantage: Don't try using one of these tools to search for a phrase or a complex search using "and" or "or." Because every search tool works differently, your complex search might result in zero hits from search tools that do not understand your query. Stick to one-word searches when using metasearch sites.

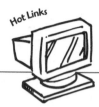

Hot Links

Engines You Can Take for a Spin

Locating useful information on the Web is often a gamble. You roll the dice with your favorite search engine and see what comes up—sometimes ending up with nothing after an hour of browsing Web page after Web page. It's cheaper than a casino, but no more productive. Using only one search tool, or using a number of search tools ineffectively, might leave you with empty pockets. So, what's the solution? Learn how to search skillfully using a few different tools by reading the "advanced" or "refine" instructions given on the search's Web site. Here are some of the biggest and best search tools—try them all and see which ones work best for you.

➤ **Yahoo!,** http://www.yahoo.com   The oldest, largest, and probably best-known Web directory.

➤ **Excite,** http://www.excite.com   One of the most popular search engines.

➤ **AltaVista,** http://www.altavista.com   Offers a wide range of advanced searching options; allows advertisers to pay to be listed first in search results.

➤ **HotBot,** http://www.hotbot.com   Reported to be the largest indexer of the Web.

➤ **GoTo,** http://www.goto.com   Companies can pay to be listed higher in the search results, which might or might not improve relevancy.

➤ **Snap,** http://www.snap.com   A Web directory supplemented by a search engine.

➤ **Looksmart,** http://www.looksmart.com   Another large Web directory.

➤ **DogPile,** http://www.dogpile.com   A metasearch that combines 13 different engines and directories.

➤ **SavvySearch,** http://www.savvysearch.com   An excellent metasearch that enables you to choose from more than 100 search tools and rank them so that results from your favorite search engines are given more importance.

Types of Web Sites

You will typically begin your ride on the information superhighway with a visit to a few search sites, and then continue on to find some favorite sites that you bookmark and visit regularly. This section explains the many different types of sites you will come across and how each of them can be used.

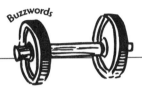

Buzzwords

Bookmark: When you "bookmark" a Web page, your computer saves the name and address of the site and keeps it in a file so that you can access it quickly at any time. Bookmarks are a great way to keep track of your favorite Web sites so that you don't have to start from scratch and search for them each time you are online.

Jump Sites: Links Galore!

Jump sites, meta sites, link sites...whatever you call them, they're often good places to start when searching the Web for information on a broad topic. Jump sites offer categorized listings of Web sites that pertain to a specific topic. They are useful when you have the time to browse a bit and see "what's out there" on your chosen topic. There are good jump sites—compiled by someone who has knowledge of the topic and cares enough to point you to the best sites—and there are bad jump sites—advertiser and traffic-driven sites that link to anyone who might put a buck in their pocket. We'll point you to lots of quality jump sites throughout this book.

Get Up

Jump Site Jump Rope

If you have a jump rope, grab it. If you don't, pretend you have one. (It's a harmless fantasy.) Each time you click to receive information or narrow your topic, get up and jump rope until the site loads.

News and Information

For some, a favorite Web news site has replaced the morning paper. And although you can't read your Web news on the train ride to work, these sites offer a convenient way to find recent news on a myriad of health and fitness topics. Jump-start your day with one of these reputable health information sites:

Reuters Health eLine

> http://publish.reutershealth.com/frame_eline.html

Consumer-oriented articles on health, diet, exercise, and disease are covered by one of the top news services in the world.

OnHealth.com

> http://www.onhealth.com

OnHealth offers daily news and in-depth reports on wellness and medicine (see Figure 2.2).

Figure 2.2

In-depth reports and regular columns make OnHealth.com worth a daily visit.

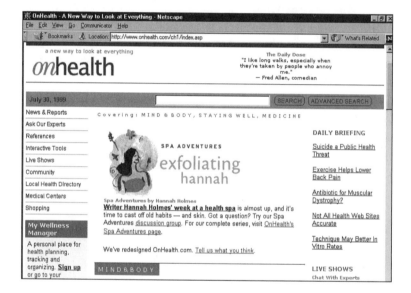

drkoop.com

> http://www.drkoop.com

Former U.S. Surgeon General C. Everett Koop provides a powerhouse site chock-full of news and other resources.

HealthCentral.com

> http://www.healthcentral.com

Read the top stories, news specials, and Dr. Dean Edell radio topics on this valuable site.

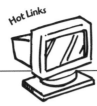

Health and Fitness at About.com

`http://home.about.com/health/`

About.com is a Web directory with a twist. Each topic in the directory has a "guide"—a real person who is an expert in the topic. The guides write articles on their topics and scour the Web for useful links. Their health and fitness section is a great place to start your surfing!

Magazines and Trade Publications

Whether you want to read back issues of your favorite magazine, use magazine archives for research, or simply check out a magazine before you subscribe, the Web can satisfy your needs. Just search for a magazine title—almost all of them have useful Web sites.

FAQs

FAQ (pronounced "fak") stands for "Frequently Asked Questions." These are Web pages that answer the public's most frequently asked questions on a specific topic. When you're searching for information on a topic you know very little about, a FAQ can be extremely useful. Many Web sites have their own FAQ, or you can try searching for your topic at The Internet FAQ Consortium, `http://www.faqs.org`.

Associations and Institutions

Government agencies, universities, consumer-education organizations, and professional associations offer tons of useful information on their Web sites. You can join an association geared toward your favorite fitness activity (how about adventure cycling at `http://www.adv-cycling.org`?), learn how to become a certified fitness professional (try the American Council on Exercise, `http://www.acefitness.org`), or learn more about a specific disease (visit the American Institute for Cancer Research, `http://www.aicr.org`).

If you don't have the specific name of an organization to search for, we suggest starting out with a "jump site" that has a category devoted to health and fitness organizations, or use a Web directory to search for your topic and browse until you find a reputable organization's Web site (look for .org, .edu, or .gov in the URL).

Personal Pages

Web surfer, beware! *Anyone* can put a Web site on the World Wide Web. Publishing a Web site with your own pictures, personal opinions, and tidbits of information is fun, inexpensive (sometimes free), and relatively simple. You don't need a lot of technical know-how and you certainly don't need to be an "expert" in anything to put up a Web site. And no one stops shady characters from claiming expertise they don't have, pretending to be doctors or nutritionists, inventing testimonials for their products, or indulging in any other fantasy at the unwary consumer's expense.

As you search for valuable health and fitness information on the Web, you'll come across many personal Web pages devoted to miracle cures, truly weird treatments, and photos of bodybuilders and fitness models (sometimes X-rated—keep your eye on the kiddies!), in addition to well-meaning, self-proclaimed "experts" who want to give you unfounded and/or unresearched advice. Some of these are really cheesy.

Storefront Sites: Sell, Sell, Sell

It is often said that "content is king" on the Internet, but "making a buck" really rules the kingdom. Search for any topic and you're bound to find myriad sites that want to sell you something. This isn't necessarily bad—especially when you're looking for the perfect book or that special piece of exercise equipment you can't find in a local store. Prices are sometimes cheaper on the Internet and the rise in popularity of "auction" sites makes it easy for you to buy something secondhand. But again, beware of the gimmicks and scams on the Web that continue to multiply. Before buying anything, read every word of this book—oh, okay, on the topics that interest you or make you want to shop—for tips on how not to get taken in.

CyberFriends: Mailing Lists, Newsgroups, Bulletin Boards, and Chat

In addition to the wealth of information you can find online, you can also find a wealth of new friends and support in your quest for a healthier lifestyle.

Finding and Using Mailing Lists

Vegetarian cooking? Seasonal affective disorder? Sports injuries? Irritable bowel syndrome? If you're looking for animated and varied discussions on any topic whatsoever, check out private mailing lists on the Internet. Topics cover everything from acne to Zoloft. The subscribers are passionate and well-informed. To subscribe to a mailing list, send an email message to a subscription address. You have to follow the list's instructions for specifics—each list has a different subscription procedure. Then you receive all the messages posted each day on the list's topic. Be prepared for plenty of email!

Mailing lists can be moderated or unmoderated. We recommend a moderated list, meaning there is a person who reads every message and forwards only the relevant posts. This cuts down on email traffic, eliminates duplicate topic postings, prevents spam, and keeps the conversation on track. In an unmoderated list, you might find yourself sifting through email hoaxes ("warnings" about computer viruses or "evidence" that certain foods are harmful for you) or personal emails from other members that should have been exchanged off the list.

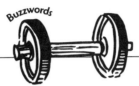

Buzzwords

Spam: An email, bulletin board, or newsgroup message that is posted repeatedly in inappropriate places. This might include unsolicited commercial email that tries to sell you something, or derogatory messages regarding lifestyle, political views, or religion. Also known as "junk email."

The following Web sites can help you find mailing lists on any topic:

➤ Liszt, `http://www.liszt.com`

➤ Publicly Accessible Mailing Lists, `http://www.neosoft.com/internet/paml`

➤ Tile.net, `http://www.tile.net/lists/`

➤ CataList, `http://www.l-soft.com/catalist.html`

➤ ONElist, `http://www.onelist.com`

➤ Topica, `http://www.topica.com`

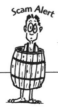

Scam Alert

Don't Answer Spam

If you get spam and it gives a "respond-to" address to get off the mailing list, don't respond! They're just trying to find out which of the email addresses they bought (or found randomly) are "live." If you respond, your email address gets used and sold over and over again. Most ISPs and online services have an email address for reporting spam. Forward unwanted and annoying spam to that address, and then delete it.

Finding and Using Newsgroups

Newsgroups, often referred to by the technical name "Usenet," are typically unmoderated and less focused than mailing lists. Messages are posted to an Usenet site and you need to revisit the site day after day to read new postings.

Newsgroups are not on the Web. They have their own interface and you need software called a "newsreader" to access them. Most browsers come with a newsreader (such as Microsoft's Outlook Express or Netscape's Messenger) which enables you to search through the thousands of newsgroups available. You don't "subscribe" to a newsgroup as you do a mailing list, so participants come and go more often than they do in mailing lists.

Some newsgroups have a core group of participants that are extremely active and helpful, so this is often a great place to go to find a real, live person who can answer your question. If you're just looking for an answer to a specific question, and you don't want to join a mailing list and discuss the topic on a regular basis, newsgroups offer an alternative. For example, you read about a new herbal remedy in a magazine and you'd like to find out more from someone who's actually used it. You might visit the `misc.health.alternative` newsgroup and pose your question. It's likely that someone participating in the newsgroup can tell you whether the herb is useful, has side effects, or is a gimmick.

The following Web sites can help you find newsgroups on any topic:

➤ DejaNews, `http://www.deja.com`

➤ Liszt, `http://www.liszt.com/news`

➤ Tile.net, `http://www.tile.net/news`

Finding and Using Bulletin Boards

Bulletin boards, also known as "message boards" and "forums," are similar to newsgroups, but are typically much smaller and more tightly focused on a single topic than newsgroups. Bulletin boards are located on Web sites, so they are easy to access—just find a good bulletin board, bookmark it, and visit regularly to post your messages or respond to others. One caveat—bulletin boards are often unmoderated, which allows for lots of spam, advertising, and unrelated conversation. Search for bulletin boards on the Web at Forum One, `http://www.forumone.com`.

If you are a member of an online service such as America Online or CompuServe, these services offer tons of bulletin boards that are not available on the Web. Just do a standard keyword search on your topic of interest and the online service points you to relevant bulletin boards.

Finding and Using Chat Rooms

Chat rooms are areas you can go to "talk" in real time with others on the Internet. You type in your message using your Web browser or chat software and it is instantly relayed to all others in your "chat room." And you receive instant responses! It's fun, it's easy, and it's addictive! More and more Web sites are offering chat rooms—some rooms are "open" all the time, so you can chat anytime there is someone else in the room. Others have scheduled chat times and topics and even experts and celebrities to answer your questions. The nature of chat doesn't allow for in-depth discussions, but it's a great place to ask questions, make friends, and gain support.

Here's the lowdown on how to chat:

➤ Online services, such as America Online, CompuServe, and Prodigy, offer the easiest access to chat rooms covering hundreds of topics. No special software is needed—just visit the health or fitness areas of these online services and you can easily find chat rooms that cater to a topic you are interested in.

➤ There are various software programs that enable you to chat over the Internet without using an online service. One such program is called IRC (Internet Relay Chat), `http://www.mirc.com`. Just download the software, install it on your computer, and then use the Liszt site at `http://liszt.com/chat/` to search through more than 37,000 chat rooms, or "channels."

➤ Web-based chats work through your standard browser. Just like a bulletin board, you visit the chat Web site, log in, and start chatting. Web-based chat rooms are typically slower, and less popular than IRC or online service chats.

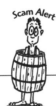

Scam Alert

Approach with Caution!

Use caution when discussing any private issues with strangers over the Internet. You don't know who these people are or how they might use your personal information. Be aware that all messages you post—to a mailing list, newsgroup, bulletin board, and sometimes even chat—are archived and kept on the Internet indefinitely. Visit a site like DejaNews and notice how people's posts are readily available for the searching. We advise not using your real name, or at least just stick to first names, and never give out your address or phone number.

25

The Least You Need to Know

➤ All search engines are not created equal, and you need to test many search tools to find the ones that work best for you.

➤ Health and fitness information on the Internet is abundant and comes in many different forms.

➤ Finding a friend for support or a forum to pose a question is as easy as a mouse click when using mailing lists, newsgroups, bulletin boards, and chat.

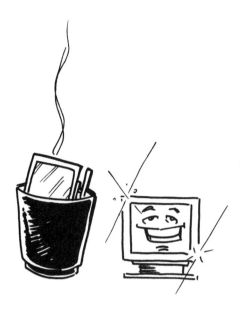

Chapter 3

Junk or Jewel? Evaluating Web Site Content and Protecting Yourself

In This Chapter

➤ Understanding the potential for online health fraud

➤ Determining the reliability of information on the Internet

➤ Protecting yourself from clever marketers

➤ Evaluating online information using the PILOT method

The Web makes it simple for just about anyone—physicians, patients, researchers, vendors, kooks, your Aunt Eleanor, or that weird neighbor who never leaves his apartment—to disseminate useful—or useless—information. It's often difficult to distinguish between reliable content and entertainment or advertising. Quick and easy access to virtually boundless health and fitness information has its benefits, but it also has serious drawbacks. Some advice can be downright harmful.

How reliable is the information you find on the Internet? That depends. It can be completely reliable and exceedingly useful, but you need to learn how to determine whether the Web site that interests you is junk or a jewel.

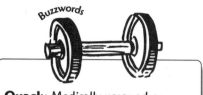

Quack: Medically unsound or promises something it doesn't deliver.

Protect Yourself from Scams

Clever marketers use the Web to make science and snake oil appear equally true. Consumers who are desperate for answers to their health or fitness problems might be easily swayed by fraudulent claims or earnest, but worthless, opinions. Protect yourself by learning about the quackery and fraud that is abundant online.

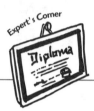

"There's some outstanding information, there's some fair information, and then there's some really dangerous, deceitful information that's deliberately put up there to market inappropriate products."

— John H. Renner, M.D., who chooses "stars and stinkers" for the Web site,
`http://www.healthscout.com/`

They Want Your Money!

The Web is full of misinformation and products that claim to perform miracles on your body. Lose 30 pounds in 30 days without diet or exercise! Restore sexual potency to teenage vigor! Turn a bald pate into a full head of curly hair! Cure cancer with the secret the medical establishment doesn't want you to know! Each year, consumers waste billions of dollars on unproven, fraudulently marketed, and sometimes unsafe health and fitness products.

You've bought them. We all have. We all hope that suddenly there will be a miracle cure, a fountain of youth, or a magic bullet to remedy all of our health concerns. But the truth is there is no secret ingredient, so don't waste your cash.

When you surf the Web for health and fitness information, keep in mind one basic fact: Companies are out there to make money. They don't know you, and most don't care about your plight. They just want your money. With e-commerce becoming more and more common, a company selling a product doesn't have to see you face-to-face or even speak to you on the phone. Con artists happily take your money right over the Internet in a completely anonymous rip-off.

"But there's a money-back guarantee!" you insist. Guess what? A scam artist is in the business of selling you with soothing, hopeful words. Who do you think enforces that money-back guarantee? They might not even be in business anymore after taking a significant amount of money from unsuspecting customers.

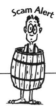

Scam Alert

It's a Jungle

Only 47 percent of 160 randomly chosen health Web sites were produced by established health and consumer-education organizations, according to a study by Interactive Solutions. The rest were operated by consumers, sellers, manufacturers, and unidentified sources. Consumers produced one out of four health sites in 1998. But how do you know that whatever is being touted actually cured one person's cancer or caused another to drop 60 pounds, or if it did, that it will work for you? You don't. If a certain product or treatment intrigues you, substantiate the evidence—don't take one person's word for anything.

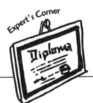

Expert's Corner

"If you find sites that make exaggerated claims about specific products, it's probably not valid information. Anything that says 'scientifically proven' without providing information about the clinical evidence is suspect. Be cautious of 'it's safe and natural' claims for products."

—Chris Hendel, Senior Researcher, *Consumer Reports on Health*

If It Sounds Too Good to Be True, It Probably Is

This is your new mantra as you surf the Web for quality health and fitness information. Ask yourself this question: If there really were a medical breakthrough, secret ingredient, or ancient remedy, would it hide in a Web site advertisement or be announced by email spam? Of course not.

You read about the many people who've had success on a certain program or with a certain product. Forget it. Anyone can say anything. Even if they're telling the truth, the diet, product, or piece of exercise equipment might have worked for a couple of people, but do you know the whole story? What else were these people doing while they took the magic fat-eliminator pill? Maybe they were dieting and exercising and that's why they lost weight. Maybe they are the product seller's in-laws. Maybe they don't even exist. Never pin your hopes for disease cure or weight loss or muscle gain on a product that sounds too good to be true, because it usually is.

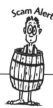

Scam Alert

Operation Cure.All

The Federal Trade Commission (FTC) launched "Operation Cure.All" in June 1999, a campaign aimed at curbing fraudulent health claims on the Internet. Operation Cure.All uses the Internet "both as a law enforcement tool to stop bogus claims for products and treatments touted as cures for various diseases and as a communication tool to provide consumers with good-quality health information," says the FTC.

The FTC got a running start by warning operators of 800 different Web sites and charging four companies with making deceptive and unsubstantiated health claims for "miracle cures" for serious illnesses. One advertised a beef-tallow arthritis cure, another shark cartilage capsules to cure cancer and AIDS/HIV, and two were magnetic therapy devices advertised to treat cancer, high blood pressure, and a wide variety of other ailments.

Can Operation Cure.All stop online health fraud? No, but it helps. As consumers get more savvy, they'll be taken in less frequently. But we suspect that the companies will also get more savvy at appealing to your emotions and hopes without breaking the letter of the law. Stay ever vigilant!

Evaluating Web Site Content: The PILOT Method

To help you PILOT your way through the friendly skies of World Wide Web health and fitness information, we've developed a method for evaluating Web site content.

This systematic approach helps you quickly weed out the truly useless information and zero in on content that can educate you and help you achieve your health and fitness goals.

P   **Purpose**

I   **Information**

L   **Links**

O   **Originator**

T   **Timeliness**

Purpose

If the site has a mission statement, read it. (It might be called "Mission," "Who Are We?," "About Us," or something similar.) If not, read the home page and analyze the site's purpose. Does it inform, persuade, sell, outrage, or entertain? Ask yourself these questions:

➤ Does the site aim to educate people with articles and/or research that inform fairly?

➤ Is the site trying to sell you something? Be especially wary if this site is the only source for this product.

➤ Is it trying to convince you that one opinion is better than another?

➤ Is the site a personal page, designed as an outlet for someone's personal health and fitness regimen?

➤ What can you tell about the site's target audience?

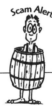

Scam Alert

Hide Your Dollars

Does the site charge a fee for information about a product or plan? Keep your wallet firmly planted in your purse or back pocket. Certainly, some reputable sites do charge a fee to cover their expenses if they offer access to large volumes of medical information, or a subscription fee for their journal or organization. But a site that wants to charge you for the greatest weight-loss discovery, or the cancer cure that the medical establishment doesn't want you to know, or an antiaging breakthrough? Hogwash.

Information

Truly useful Web sites offer valuable information. That means more than advertising or splashy graphics. Be aware that advertising might be cleverly disguised as an article or "scientific research." The bottom line: If the site is selling anything, ask yourself how that might influence the content. (That's not to say all sellers are underhanded and devious, waiting to steal your hard-earned cash, but some of them are, and it's best to approach them all with healthy suspicion.) Keep the following in mind:

➤ Does the information further your knowledge of health and fitness issues?

➤ Is the content fact, supported by documented research, credible sources, or authoritative references?

➤ Are undocumented case histories used as "proof" to substantiate claims?

➤ Is the content opinion, and if so, whose opinion is it, and how credible is the opinion holder?

➤ Is the content propaganda, designed to persuade you and appeal to your emotions? If so, resist.

➤ If the site is selling a product, plan, or service, how much is the content biased toward what's being sold?

➤ Has the site won any awards? If so, from whom?

➤ Beware of sites that say "only" and "best." Reputable sites do not claim to be the sole source of information on a topic and do not disrespect other credible sources of knowledge.

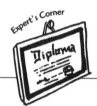

Expert's Corner

"Trying to get health information from the Internet is like drinking from a fire hose, and you don't even know what the source of the water is."

—Mary Jo Deering, director of health communication and telehealth for the Department of Health and Human Services

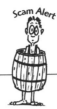

Check the Company

If you do decide to purchase a product online, phone the company first. Ask about the procedure for getting a refund. Find out where the company is located, and contact the Better Business Bureau to see whether there have been complaints. If the company does not give an address, do not order.

Links

The best sites want to inform you and are happy to recommend additional Web sites to further your knowledge in that topic or related topics.

➤ The more, the merrier—lots of links make for a great Web resource.

➤ Are the selected links recommended, related, and reliable sites? Random sites that run the gamut from credible to incredible might be fun on a rainy afternoon, but are frustrating when you're looking for the best information swiftly.

➤ Look for sites that organize their links into helpful categories, or better yet, include a rating and/or review.

➤ Be sure the links are up to date—if you click on a few and they're "dead" (no longer operational), move on to another site.

➤ Does the site have an "add your own link" feature or a long list of banners, sometimes unrelated to the topic? These serve only to drive more traffic to the Web site—they don't further your education/research of your topic.

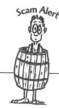

Scam Alert

Trust Your Gut

If a site is poorly organized and unattractive, that might be a major clue that the creator of the site is not professional enough to design a nice-looking, user-friendly Web page. Likewise, if the site is riddled with numerous colors, blinking words, exclamation points, or flashing graphics to the point that it's difficult to discern the content, those are sometimes indicators of quack sites. These elements don't prove that the site was put up by a bunch of lowlifes snickering in their basement or a "loony toon" who can't get anyone else to listen, but do you really want to trust this person with your health decisions? User experience—the organization, flow, and overall "feel" of the site—should be a factor in your evaluation.

Originator

Before you take any advice found on the Internet, determine who is responsible for the information. Is this readily apparent on the Web site? Best bets for sound health and fitness information are consumer advocacy groups, health professional organizations, well-known hospitals, and government- and university-sponsored sites.

➤ Who is responsible for the information? Look for an individual's name or the name of an organization.

➤ If the originator is an organization, what does it stand for?

➤ If the originator is a person, what are his or her credentials, occupation, and affiliation? Does the author have the experience and authority to provide this info?

➤ Is the originator affiliated with a specific product or program? Is the site financially tied to a commercial venture through sponsorship, advertising, or underwriting? (If so, there still might be great information on the site if it passes the rest of our test, but take "proof" that a certain product is the best with many grains of salt.)

➤ Can you contact the originator by email or other means? The most reputable organizations/site publishers disclose full addresses and phone numbers so that they can be contacted.

➤ Don't trust any physician or health guru who diagnoses, treats, or prescribes online.

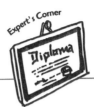

Expert's Corner

"We hope Americans continue to use the Internet for truthful information, but we also want them to have their antennas up to be careful about those claims that are exaggerated."

—Jodie Bernstein, director of the FTC's Bureau of Consumer Protection

Timeliness

Depending on the topic you are looking into exploring, the information should not be more than a few years old. Medical information should be more current. For example, a medical site with out-of-date information could list a drug as safe even though it has recently been found to cause dangerous side effects; or a site might tout a treatment as effective when it is now considered worthless. With health and fitness being a dynamic, constantly researched field, more frequent updates are better.

➤ Is the information current? Look for dates in bylines of articles or look for current issues on publication Web sites.

➤ How often is the site updated? Ideally, a site with time-sensitive health information should be updated daily, weekly, or monthly.

➤ If the information has not been updated recently, is this material that you can trust not to go out of date?

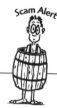

Email Health Hoaxes

We don't know what kind of people get their kicks by starting email health scares, but they've come up with some doozies. Here's the truth about a few common ones:

➤ Waterproof sunscreen will not make your children go blind.

➤ Antiperspirants do not cause breast cancer.

➤ Aspartame does not cause multiple sclerosis or lupus.

➤ HIV-infected needles are not being found in telephone coin returns or movie theaters.

➤ Tampons do not contain asbestos.

➤ Shampoo does not cause cancer.

If you want to check out these or any other hair-raising health warnings you might read on the Internet, Dr. Dean Edell has a bunch of reports at `http://www.healthcentral.com`. Click **Hot Topics**, and then **Internet Hoax Watch**.

If you get an email that warns you about some awful health consequence of an innocuous product or ordinary behavior, just delete it, even if it comes from your high-school sweetheart. And please, when it implores you to send it to your entire mailing list (and it will), don't! Especially when it has a lot of exclamation points!!!!!!

Start Here

If you're new to searching out health information on the Web, you want to start with a credible site that screens its links. That way you can depend on the value of the information you're getting while you learn to evaluate the sites yourself. Here's a good place to start.

Healthfinder

`http://www.healthfinder.gov`

This site is "a free gateway to reliable consumer health and human services information" developed by the U.S. Department of Health and Human Services. Healthfinder (see Figure 3.1) leads you to selected online publications, clearinghouses, databases, Web sites, support and self-help groups, government agencies, and not-for-profit organizations, all selected for their reliable information. 3,200 links in all! No advertising, no sales, no commercial links. This is a great starting place for information on any general health topic.

And if you wish this chapter were longer because you want to learn more about online health fraud, check out

`http://www.healthfinder.gov/smartchoices/fraud/quack.htm`, which links to fraud alert articles on topics as varied as dieting, food labels, home medical equipment, and herbal remedies.

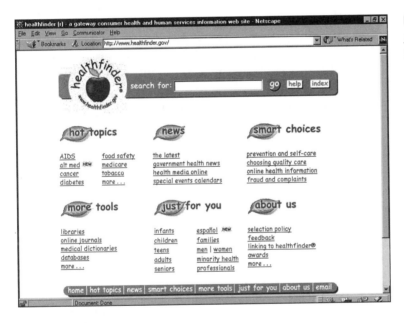

Figure 3.1

Healthfinder is a gateway to screened health sites.

Evaluation Grad School

After you understand the basics of how to evaluate a health Web site using our PILOT Method, you might want to learn more about the potential for fraud and the tools to slash your way through them. If you want to delve deeper, here are your professors:

Quackwatch

`http://www.quackwatch.com/`

This enormous site, "Your Guide to Health Fraud, Quackery, and Intelligent Decisions," is operated by Stephen Barrett, M.D., who is on a crusade to "combat health-related frauds, myths, fads, and fallacies," especially on the Internet. More than 100 articles are listed under Questionable Products, Services, and Theories, and that's just part of the site. Check it out.

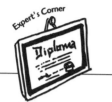

"The Internet is a veritable mine-field of false and misleading claims."

—Bruce Silverglade, Center for Science in the Public Interest, http://www.cspinet.org/

Locating and Evaluating Health Information on the Internet

http://imt.net/~randolfi/HealthyWebs.html

Scroll past the links to find an excellent article, "Evaluating Health/Medical Information on the Internet." It's written in an academic rather than consumer-friendly style (this *is* graduate school), but the information is clear. Afterwards, take a look at the links to other sites about evaluating health and medical Web sites. The list is maintained by Ernesto (Ernie) A. Randolfi, Ph.D., associate professor at Montana State University, Billings.

How to Understand and Interpret Food and Health-Related Scientific Studies

http://ificinfo.health.org/brochure/ificrevu.htm.

If you're ready to tackle the challenge of how to be an educated reader of the research, this article introduces you gently, defines all the terms you need, and even tells you how to question the experts. The information is from the International Food Information Council.

The Least You Need to Know

➤ Clever marketers can deceive you with a well-designed Web site. Don't be taken in by sites that claim to offer credible content, but are really out to capture your cash.

➤ Use the PILOT method to evaluate a Web site: Purpose, Information, Links, Originator, and Timeliness.

➤ When considering health and fitness recommendations found online, search for evidence to back up a claim. If you can't find any site that corroborates the information, it's probably best left alone.

Part 2

Working Out on the Web

A few generations ago, exercise used to be a regular part of daily life. People walked around town, climbed stairs, grew their own vegetables, and did housework with brooms, mops, and elbow grease. Kids swam, ran, skated, jumped rope, and played tag. But now it's too easy not to exercise, so we must schedule and make time for it.

If you don't yet have an exercise habit, these chapters help you use the Internet to start one. And if you are active already, we introduce you to fresh options, workout information, tips, and new friends.

Exercise isn't about being skinny. It's about being happy, confident, energetic, and healthy. So, lace up your walking shoes and join us as we show you how to develop your own personal fitness program and use Internet resources to make the most of your exercise regimen.

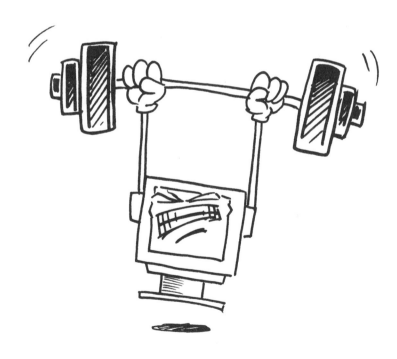

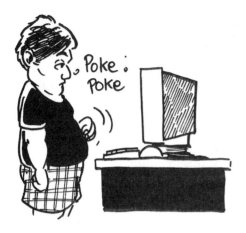

Chapter 4

Developing Your Personal Fitness Program

In This Chapter

➤ Setting realistic personal goals

➤ Developing a fitness program you can stick to for life

➤ Using online tools to evaluate your fitness level

➤ Creating a program that will help you reach your goals

If you'd rather surf the Web than walk the park, let the Internet motivate and educate you with the extraordinary resources available online. You can take fitness-assessment tests (yes, you have to leave the computer for a few minutes), get help setting your goals, and find personalized tips for setting up a plan that will work for you. Get your sneakers ready, and let this chapter help you get started.

If you're already a committed exerciser, congratulations! Our tips here help you evaluate the results of your program and decide your next steps.

How Fit Are You?

If you haven't been exercising regularly, it's useful to determine your current level of health and fitness before you take off running (or walking). If you are under 35 and have no health problems that might interfere, you can begin an exercise program this

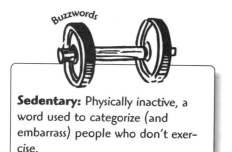

Buzzwords

Sedentary: Physically inactive, a word used to categorize (and embarrass) people who don't exercise.

minute. However, if you are over 35, have health problems, or have been sedentary for years, check in with your physician before beginning an exercise program. Your doctor will first applaud your new resolution. Then after you take a bow, he or she might want to perform a few tests, such as a blood-pressure check, and discuss any limitations you might have. After you've got the go-ahead, you can do some tests of your own to pinpoint where you need to focus your fitness efforts.

Determining Your Fitness Level

These are the four basic components you need to evaluate to determine your fitness level:

➤ **Cardiovascular (aerobic) fitness**   How effectively do your heart and lungs deliver blood and oxygen throughout your body? Do you have the stamina to do the activities you enjoy?

➤ **Muscle strength**   How strong are your muscles? How well will they protect your joints and bones and let you perform daily tasks as you age?

➤ **Flexibility**   How flexible are you? The range of motion of your joints decreases as you age, or when you become sedentary, and this eventually can limit everyday abilities such as bending or reaching. A regular stretching program can keep your muscles loose and your joints flexible.

➤ **Body composition**   What percentage of your weight is fat? Do you carry too much body fat compared to lean tissue? Does the amount of body fat interfere with your health, activities, or quality of life?

Fitness testing is useful both before beginning your personal exercise program and to evaluate your progress. When you see that you are inching closer to your fitness goals, you stay motivated. Repeat your fitness tests every two to three months to track fitness gains and increase your motivation.

Fitness Testing Information Online

There are tests that you can do in the privacy of your own home to evaluate these four elements of fitness. However, be aware that your results are only general indications of your fitness level—you might not be doing the test exactly right, or there might be errors in the calculation of results. Also, the online test might not take into account other variables, such as whether you're exercising with asthma, rehabilitating from a back injury, or doing physical work in your daily life. So, use the fitness tests, but take them as indicators, not gospel. Check out the following sites for details on fitness testing.

"Developing Your Fitness Program" by the American Medical Association

http://www.ama-assn.org/insight/gen_hlth/trainer/index.htm

Read the AMA's excellent advice on the benefits of physical activity, and then click **Fitness Assessment Questionnaire** for detailed instructions on how to perform various fitness tests. You can do the basic self-evaluation (A) or get up and perform physical tests for the more comprehensive assessment (B), which we recommend (see Figure 4.1).

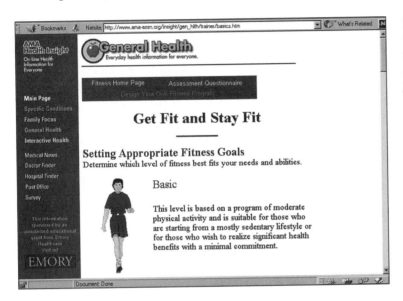

Figure 4.1

The AMA explains how to test your fitness level and design your own fitness program.

Shape Up America Fitness Club Assessment

http://www.shapeup.org/fitness/assess/fset2.htm

You get your choice of fitness tests here: PAR-Q test for readiness for physical activity, Activity Level Assessment to evaluate your present level of activity, Flexibility Test to measure range of movement, Muscular Strength and Endurance Test for the upper body, and two tests for aerobic fitness.

Rob Wood's Fitness Testing Site

http://fitness.testing.8m.com

Exercise physiologist Dr. Robert Wood offers a great list of fitness tests, from basic tests you can do at home to advanced tests that require specific equipment. The "Guide to: physical fitness testing" offers information on the benefits of testing, and how to select, conduct, and interpret fitness tests. Although a lot of the information

43

on this site is geared toward coaches and athletes, just about anyone can gain valuable insight into fitness testing techniques and advantages.

Phantom Chair Assessment Test

Here's an easy way to assess the strength of your quadriceps, the large muscles of the front of the thighs that power so many physical activities. Stand with your back against a wall, and slide down, keeping your back against the wall and walking your feet away from the wall. Keep your feet right under your knees. When your thighs are almost parallel to the floor, stop and count the number of seconds you can "sit" there before the burning in your thighs makes you get up. After you start a regular exercise program, repeat this test once a month to see how your thigh strength improves.

Setting Reachable Goals

After determining where your fitness level *is*, your next step is determining where your fitness level *should* be. Whether you want to lose weight, gain muscle, or run a 10K, you need a specific plan to get you there: a set of realistic goals.

A vague ("get in shape") or unrealistic ("lose 25 pounds before my class reunion in three weeks") goal can be counterproductive and demoralizing. If you expect too much and you don't achieve it, you're more likely to quit. Begin by writing down the final result you hope to achieve. Let's say you're starting a walking program. You can walk only two miles in an hour, and you'd like to increase your walking speed to 4mph—and add some hills.

Next, give yourself a realistic time frame and set a goal to mark the achievement of half of your goal—let's say achieving a walk of 3 miles in one hour, and adding one hill, after walking for two months. Finally, cut your halfway goal in half again to give yourself a short-term goal of walking 2.5 miles in an hour over the next four weeks.

You can use a similar system, even when your goals are not quantifiable by numbers. Want to gain muscle and lose fat? You can set your goals in terms of the amount of weight you can lift, or the dress size you wear.

After you've got your goals in writing, think of them as a ladder—then climb it!

Developing Your Fitness Program

You've tested your fitness level and set your goals. Are you ready to jam to the gym and get going? Not yet! Your next step is to develop a program that fits your lifestyle and helps you achieve your goals.

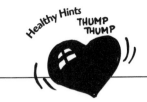

Healthy Hints

Goal Number One

An excellent goal is simply to "show up" to your chosen exercise session every day!

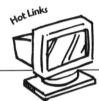

Hot Links

"Easing into Exercise" by Joan Price

http://www.joanprice.com

Joan specializes in helping nonexercisers get started. Here she helps you take your first steps. Scroll down to a list of helpful articles and excerpts from her book *Joan Price Says, Yes, You CAN Get in Shape!* Be sure to read "Making Fitness Happen" and "Yes, You CAN! Tips for Sticking to Your Exercise Program" for motivation and helpful hints.

If you're new to exercise, we recommend setting up a session with a personal fitness trainer. A fitness trainer can evaluate your fitness level and also talk with you about your personal style. What type of activities do you enjoy? How can you make those activities work for you to achieve your goals? Certified trainers can be found in your Yellow Pages, through your doctor, through a local health club, and even on the Internet. For more information, please read Chapter 7, "Personal Trainers: Finding One That's Right for You."

Burn Calories, Don't Eat Them

You need a break—your energy has crashed. Plan A: You reach for coffee and doughnuts to give yourself a little rush. But if you react to the combination of caffeine, sugar, flour, and fat that these foods contain as most of us do, this just ensures that your energy level will take a dive again in a couple of hours. A better idea is Plan B: "Just say no" to the pastries and caffeine, put on comfortable shoes, and push your tired body out your door. Walk around the block as briskly as possible. If going outside is not an option, stride through your house or office. You'll energize physically and mentally, and do better thinking when you get back. At a 4mph pace, you can burn 100 calories in 15 minutes. (But if you stick to plan A, you can *eat* 500 calories in 15 minutes!)

Use the Three Components of Fitness: Aerobics, Strength Training, and Stretching

When we talked about fitness assessment, we included tests for cardiovascular fitness, strength, and flexibility. A solid and effective fitness program increases all three by including aerobic activity, muscle-strengthening exercises, and stretching. (In case you're wondering about the fourth assessment—body composition—by doing aerobics and strength training, you increase your lean muscle and decrease your body fat. It all works together.)

For more information on the elements of fitness, as well as tips on improving each element, check out "Fitness Basics" from the Fitness Files at http://rcc.webpoint.com/fitness/fitbasic.htm.

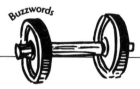

Aerobic: Aerobic means "in the presence of oxygen." Aerobic exercise is any activity that increases your respiratory rate and increases the capacity of the heart-lung system to deliver oxygen throughout the body. In practical terms, aerobic exercise is any rhythmic exercise using the large muscles that increases your heart rate.

Create a Realistic Plan and Stick to It!

Just like your goals, your fitness program must be realistic. Choose a time and a place for exercise that you can stick with for the long haul. For example, trying to tell yourself to stop at the gym every night after work when you are exhausted and really a morning person does not make sense. Find a way to fit your exercise in before breakfast. Likewise, if you can't open both eyes at the same time until after 9:00 a.m., don't sign up for the 7:30 a.m. aerobics class!

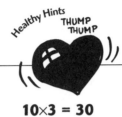

10×3 = 30

We used to think that we had to exercise for 20 to 30 minutes or more for it to "count." But several research studies now support that we get almost the same health and weight-loss benefits from several short exercise sessions throughout the day. If you're a beginner and you can't imagine lasting for 30 minutes, do 10 minutes at three different times, and the benefits are almost equivalent to doing the whole 30 minutes at once. That's good news!

Joining a Health Club Versus Working Out at Home

Joining a health club puts a dollar value on your workout time. The simple fact that money has been spent on a membership is enough to drive some people into regular workouts. Some people love the camaraderie of a health club. You can join with a friend, or make new friends who inspire you to meet them there day after day and share your ups and downs. For others, it's the atmosphere of a health club that keeps them coming back. The minute you step in the door, you've made the commitment to exercise for that day. Anything we say about health clubs, by the way, applies equally to exercise programs at your local YMCA, Jewish Community Center, or Parks and Rec.

If you decide a health club or other program is the best option for your fitness program, choose one that is convenient—you're not as likely to skip your workout if you drive right by the gym on your way to and from work.

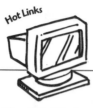

HealthClubs.com

`http://www.healthclubs.com`

To begin your search for a health club, check out this excellent site brought to you by the International Health, Racquet & Sportsclub Association. If you're not sure a health club is for you, or if you are sure and you could use help choosing one, HealthClubs.com offers terrific tips on how to choose a club, as well as providing a searchable directory that lets you search for a health club based on more than 30 service criteria. After you've found a club near you, the site provides a map and details all of the club's facilities. The service also links you to the club's official Web site, if the club has one.

Can you use the World Wide Web to choose a local health club? Maybe. Some large chains such as 24-Hour Fitness (`http://www.24hourfitness.com`) or Gold's Gym (`http://www.goldsgym.com`), and small "families" of clubs such as Baltimore's Brick Bodies (`http://www.brickbodies.com`) have their own Web sites with information about their programs, locations, and fitness in general (see Figure 4.2). Some local clubs might also have Web sites, including membership information, class schedules, and special events. But not all fitness clubs have a presence in cyberspace, so there might be a perfectly wonderful club close to your home or work that you'll only find in your local Yellow Pages.

Maybe you don't have a gym close by, or you don't want to pay the fees, or you just like the privacy of exercising in your own space. Working out at home can be easy and effective. But although it is convenient, exercising at home might not be the best choice for you. Ask yourself these important questions:

➤ Will your spouse/roommate/children be supportive of your scheduled workout time? Can you be sure they won't interrupt you?

➤ Are you motivated enough to get your sneakers on and exercise when there is a perfectly good television just waiting to be watched? Do you have the discipline to exercise alone at regularly scheduled times?

➤ Do you know how to exercise properly? Do you have videos that show you safety precautions? Are you fully aware of the proper techniques in using your home fitness equipment?

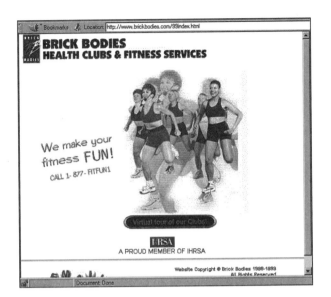

Figure 4.2
The Brick Bodies Web site offers virtual tours of their clubs, as well as programming, product, and fitness information.

Using Software to Track Your Progress

Now that you've determined your fitness level, set your goals, and decided when, where, and how you want to work out, your next step is to get started and keep track of your progress. Once again, your computer can be a valuable fitness tool by taking advantage of software tracking programs. These programs keep detailed records of your workouts and create graphs and reports to show your progress. Try a search on "fitness software" at your favorite search engine site, or try one of the following sites.

Pro Track 99 by Dakota Fit Software

```
http://www.dakotafit.com
```

This software package keeps track of your workouts, personal measurements, and nutritional information and lets you view, print, and analyze this information with graphs and reports on your computer.

CrossTrak

```
http://www.crosstrak.com
```

"CrossTrak was designed to allow athletes of all levels to quickly and easily log their workouts, monitor performance, and communicate training data with people around the globe." And this software is free!

Life Form

http://www.fitnesoft.com

Life Form helps you track health information, medical history, food, exercise, measurements, chemistry, and how you feel on a given day. Create graphs and reports to view your progress.

Online Tools to Help You Succeed

You can also use training logs that are built right into the Web. These programs are simple to use—you just visit a Web site and you don't have to download any software. These tools can be especially useful for those who travel frequently—you have access to your workout information as long as you have access to a computer! Visit one of these Web sites to log your fitness program:

ActiveLog

http://www.activelog.com

Just choose a username and password and begin logging your fitness activities. It's free and you can use the daily planner to create a schedule of future workouts or view reports and graphs of previous workouts (see Figure 4.3).

Figure 4.3

ActiveLog allows you to schedule and log your workouts online and create graphs and reports to track your progress.

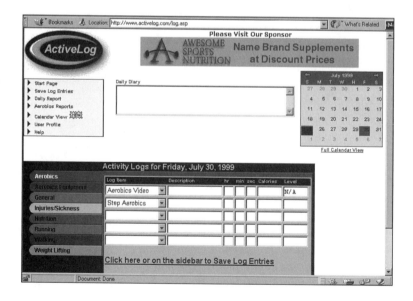

Workoutlog.com

```
http://www.workoutlog.com
```

Record your workout data, use graphs to measure your workout progress, and generate workout templates to take to the gym. You're offered a free 10-day trial, and it's only $19.95 per year after that.

Finding Workout Programs Online: Advantages and Disadvantages

You can find many types of workout regimens online. The workouts you find might inspire you to try a new activity, teach you an innovative method of exercising, or put a spark in an old, tired routine by adding different exercises. But, as you know, not every exercise program is right for every person—your program has to fit your personal goals, fitness level, and lifestyle. So, you need to inspect and personalize the program you find.

When you find a workout program online, be sure to first evaluate the site using our PILOT method. Be sure to determine the purpose of that particular program. If your goal is to train for a marathon and you're looking at a fitness program designed for bodybuilding, it's not going to work. If you're used to doing five step classes a week, a program for beginners is a waste of your time.

Start Here: Sites to Help You Develop Your Fitness Program

Searching for fitness programs on the Web can be a little tricky. You need to do some extensive searching and evaluating to find sites that provide solid recommendations. Here are some starting points for designing your program. Scout around, adapt, and tweak what you find here until you've got exactly what you want.

The Fitness Plan from The Internet's Fitness Resource

```
http://www.netsweat.com/fitplan.html
```

In addition to offering a huge jump site, the Internet's Fitness Resource offers the "basics" to developing a fitness program and points you to sites that give quality advice.

FitnessLink's 30-Minute Fat-Burning Circuit Workout

http://www.fitnesslink.com/exercise/circuit.htm

Shannon's FitnessLink site offers a circuit-type workout—you move quickly from light weight training at high repetitions to aerobic work, and back to weight training. This method builds aerobic and muscular endurance and keeps you from getting bored.

Cory Everson's Guide to Working Out

http://www.coryeverson.com

From the main page, just click **Let's Get Busy** and then select **Guide to Working Out**. Fitness guru and six-time Ms. Olympia Cory Everson offers beginner, intermediate, and advanced workout programs, as well as workouts for sports, rehab, and special needs.

The Least You Need to Know

➤ Testing your own fitness level helps you find out where you are and where you want to be, as well as measure your success as you get closer to your goals.

➤ An effective fitness program should be targeted to your goals and should include aerobic, muscle-strengthening, and stretching activities.

➤ You can find abundant information about health clubs online.

➤ Great Web sites that help you find a core training program that you can customize to meet your needs abound online.

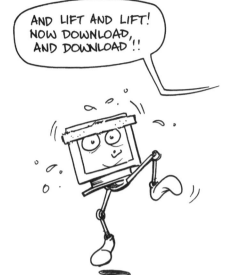

AND LIFT AND LIFT!
NOW DOWNLOAD,
AND DOWNLOAD!!

Chapter 5

Aerobics: Raising Your Heart Rate Online

> ## In This Chapter
>
> ➤ Why you need to include aerobic activity in your fitness program
>
> ➤ Determining how long and how often you need to exercise aerobically
>
> ➤ Finding information online about a variety of aerobic activities

Aerobics is much more than jumping up and down—in fact, you don't have to jump at all to do it. Do you have a favorite aerobic activity? If so, you can learn more about improving your technique, read articles about your activity of choice, and find other aficionados online. If you're dissatisfied with your aerobic routine, you can pep it up or change it entirely. And even if your aerobic routine has never progressed beyond wishful thinking, you can find an activity you'd enjoy and get all the information online that you need to get started.

This chapter explains what aerobic activity is, why you need it, and how much you need, and points you to sites where you can learn about many different options.

What Is Aerobic Activity?

You might hear the word "aerobics" and immediately picture Jane Fonda in her legwarmers a couple of decades ago, bouncing and stretching her way through an aerobic-dance workout video. But aerobic activity is much, much more than aerobic dance. And even aerobic dance has changed dramatically since the days of Jane's windmills and jumping jacks.

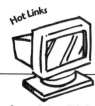

Aerobics FAQ

http://www.turnstep.com/Faq/
faq.html

Sensible answers to the most frequently asked questions about aerobic exercise can be found here.

Aerobic exercise is any activity that increases your heart rate and breathing and makes you move rhythmically and continually for a period of time. It might be biking, swimming, or running, and it might be raking leaves, mowing the lawn, or swing dancing.

Why Do You Need Aerobic Activity?

Aerobic activity is essential for a healthy heart; and it plays a major factor in weight loss and control, stress reduction, and disease prevention.

Go for the (Calorie) Burn

The magic number is 1,500 to 2,000 calories a week. No, don't eat them—burn them. A Harvard alumni study showed increased health benefits and decreased risk of cardiovascular disease in people who exercised off 1,500 to 2,000 calories weekly—regardless of what kind of exercise they did. That comes to just 30 to 60 minutes a day, most days of the week, of moderate-intensity exercise—or less time if you go for higher intensity.

Cardiovascular Health

Your seven-year-old son drags you outside to play a rousing game of soccer. You're huffing and puffing around the yard. He promptly whips you 10 to nothing.

Don't let this happen to you! Aerobic activity keeps you young and allows you to enjoy life to the fullest by making your heart stronger. As your heart muscle becomes more efficient, a larger amount of blood can be pumped with each stroke and fewer strokes are needed, lessening the workload on your heart (this is why a fit person has a lower resting heart rate than an unfit person does). If you're aerobically fit, you have more energy and reduce your risk for major diseases such as hypertension, heart disease, and stroke.

Weight Loss/Control

Aerobic activity helps you to lose or maintain weight by burning calories that would otherwise be stored as fat. This doesn't mean you've got a free ticket to eat more, but you can certainly lose weight *and* enjoy a healthy and varied diet—without going hungry. Aerobic activity acts as an appetite suppressant on the body and boosts your metabolism, keeping your body burning extra calories for hours after you've completed your exercise.

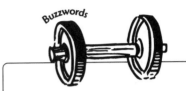

Resting Heart Rate: The number of beats per minute your heart beats at rest. The lower the number, the more efficient your heart.

Curious about how many calories you burn during your favorite activity? Try the Fitness Partner Connection Jumpsite's Activity Calorie Calculator at `http://www.primusweb.com/fitnesspartner/jumpsite/calculat.htm`. This incredibly useful tool tells you how many calories you burn per minute for 158 activities.

Stress Reduction: Exercise Makes You Feel Good!

Our bodies react to any type of stress as if it were danger, triggering the "fight or flight" response, which produces adrenaline and tenses our muscles for combat. But when there is no combat, we end up with lots of unspent energy in the form of tight, aching muscles, headaches, and even stomach problems. Exercise allows us to release that unspent energy, diffusing pent-up anger and releasing muscle tension.

Exercise can also give you a high! Maybe you've heard of endorphins—those chemicals that send good feelings radiating throughout your body. When you engage in vigorous exercise, your body responds by releasing endorphins and elevating your mood—often referred to as a "runner's high."

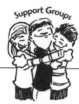

Finding a Fitness Community

Hot debates, timely conversations, and answers to your exercise questions can be found in the many online mailing lists, newsgroups, bulletin boards, and chat rooms online. If you're looking to join a community of fitness-minded people, here are a few places to start:

➤ **Fit-L mailing list** `http://maelstrom.stjohns.edu/archives/fit-l.html`

➤ `misc.fitness.aerobics newsgroup`

➤ **FitnessLink's Fitness Forum bulletin board** `http://www.fitnesslink.com/forum/`

➤ **Fitness Chat at About.com** `http://home.about. com/health/fitness/chat.htm`

How Often, How Long, How Hard?

What is the ideal weekly aerobic workout? Opinions differ, but it is generally accepted that a minimum of 30 minutes of aerobic exercise, three days a week, improves stamina, fitness level, energy, and health. Advanced exercisers might be comfortable doing more. Beginners might need to exercise in shorter sessions repeated more frequently, such as 10-minute workouts, three times a day.

A constant source of debate in the fitness community is the question of how long and how hard. Does exercising at a lower heart rate for a longer period of time put you in a "fat-burning zone"? Or is vigorous exercise the best way to go?

If your goal is general heart health and weight loss or maintenance, the answer is that it doesn't really matter. Although vigorous exercise burns more calories per minute than an easier workout, an extra 15 or 30 minutes at an easier pace allows you to more than make up the difference. If you don't have much time to work out, you might try more vigorous exercise for shorter periods. If you are a beginner, you want to start out slowly and keep your workouts in the "long and easy" category.

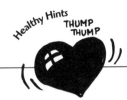

Take Time to Rest

Be careful not to exercise to exhaustion or pain. Rather than getting fit faster, you risk fatigue, ache, burnout, and injury. Schedule your vigorous aerobic workouts every other day to give your legs time to rest and strengthen.

Put Away That Magazine! Understanding Intensity

Are you one of those people who covers up the display on the treadmill with a magazine so you don't have to see how many minutes you have left to go? Instead of distracting yourself and hoping the time goes by quickly, try using the display to your advantage. Modern exercise equipment has the capability to tell you how fast you are going and how many calories you are burning, and some can even read your heart rate—all of these are tools you can use to monitor your intensity and challenge yourself for a better workout.

Intensity is how hard you are exercising. It's important to take notice of how hard you are working by checking your heart rate and perceived exertion. If you're working too hard, you might be missing out on the heart-strengthening and fat-loss benefits of aerobic activity and risking exhaustion and stress. If you're not working hard enough, you might be wasting your precious exercise time.

➤ **Calculating your target heart rate**   Subtract your age from 220. This is your maximum heart rate (MHR). Now multiply your MHR by 0.65 and 0.85 to get a range of 65% to 85% of your MHR. This is your target heart rate range in beats per minute. You want to stay within this range for an effective workout. To determine whether you're in that range during exercise, use a heart rate monitor, or simply check your pulse. Count your pulse for 6 seconds and multiply by 10 to get your beats per minute. If you're not interested in the math, try FitnessLink's Target Heart Rate Calculator at http://www.fitnesslink.com/cgi-bin/heart_rate/heart_rate.cgi.

The JanaTrains Web site has an informative article explaining heart rate ranges and the benefits of monitoring your heart rate—http://www.janatrains.com/ebzhrm.htm.

➤ **Checking your perceived exertion**   On a scale of zero to ten, how hard do you feel you're exercising? Zero would be lying on the couch doing the remote control boogie, and ten would be sucking wind after an all-out sprint.

You don't want to be at either end of the spectrum when you exercise. Keep your intensity at level four or five. You should be able to talk, but not sing a song. You should be breathing faster than normal, but not gasping for air. You might sometimes see exertion scales that go from one to 17.

You can read more about how and why to use perceived exertion, and take a look at a perceived exertion scale, on the American Council on Exercise Web site at `http://www.acefitness.org/fitfacts/ff/26.html` (see Figure 5.1).

Figure 5.1

The American Council on Exercise advises you to monitor your Rate of Perceived Exertion.

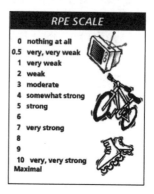

We don't mean that you have to stop in the middle of a challenging game of basketball with your buddies to check your heart rate—but if you get in the habit of monitoring your intensity when you are exercising alone, you'll come to know how you feel when you are working hard enough.

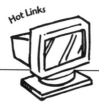

Hot Links

Fitness Partner Connection Jumpsite!

`http://www.primusweb.com/fitnesspartner/`

This site is chock-full of links to fitness information: fitness activities, mind/body, weight management, health, nutrition, kids' fitness, online publications, fitness products, and more. The Jumpsite also offers bulletin boards, a calorie calculator, and a library of excellent articles.

Types of Aerobic Activity: Finding Info Online

If you're interested in one particular type of aerobic exercise, you can find everything from online magazines and jump sites to bulletin boards and question-and-answer forums. And if you're looking to expand your exercise repertoire, do a little surfing to see whether one of the following activities is for you.

Walking

Walking Club

```
http://www.women.com/clubs/walking.html
```

"Whether you've been an avid walker for years and you want to talk about the finer points of your stride or you're new to the walking world and looking for advice, the Walking Club is the place for you to find—and share—resources."

Walking Technique and Form

```
http://www.walkingconnection.com/Walking_Technique_Form.html
```

You think you know how to walk, right? Well, just in case, this Web site details proper body alignment and fitness walking technique.

Racewalk

```
http://www.racewalk.com
```

The official racewalking Web site provides "all the information you need to start and improve your walking program, whether for competition or fitness."

Inline Skating

Skating.com: The Skater's Online Magazine

```
http://www.skating.com
```

Information on ice and inline skating.

Rollerblade.com

```
http://www.rollerblade.com
```

This sleek site gives you a 10-week workout, calorie-burning chart, skate recommendations, bulletin boards, top 10 places in the U.S. to skate, and tons of other rollerblading essentials (see Figure 5.2).

Figure 5.2

Rollerblade.com points out the fitness benefits of inline skating.

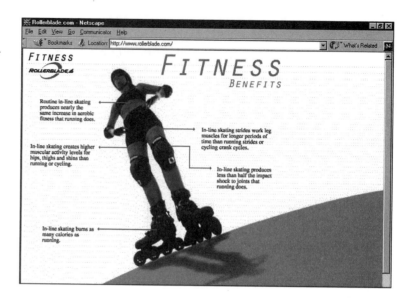

Running

NewRunner.com

http://www.newrunner.com

Brought to you by *Runner's World Magazine*, this site provides all the motivation you need to start a running program. We especially like the "Lame Excuse of the Week."

Cool Running

http://www.coolrunning.com

This site is stuffed with training tips, marathon news, running events, and running clubs.

Tennis/Squash

TennisLinks.com

http://www.tennislinks.com

This site is a great place to start with tons of links to everything tennis.

Internet Squash Federation

http://www.squash.org

Equipment, rankings, rules, tournaments, chat, newsletter, and more. "The only Internet Squash site officially sanctioned by the World Squash Federation."

Swimming

SwimInfo

http://www.swiminfo.com

So much swimming info that you won't have time to swim (see Figure 5.3)!

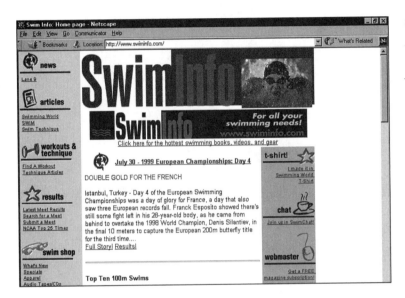

Figure 5.3

SwimInfo offers news, articles, workouts, shopping, swim meet results, and chat for swimming enthusiasts.

Swim 2000

http://www.swim2000.com

Books, videos, goggles, suits, world records, links, and swimming FAQ—it's all here at Swim 2000. You can even have weekly swimming workouts delivered to your email box!

Cycling

Bicycling Magazine Online

http://www.bicyclingmagazine.com

With informative features such as "The Principles of Pedaling" and "How Cycling Fights Aging," this is a must-see site for anyone interested in cycling. Don't forget to visit the BikeFinder to help you choose the perfect bike.

Cyber Cyclery: Internet Bicycling Hub

http://cycling.org/

Talk with other cyclists through mailing lists and bulletin boards, or use their bike shop directory, classifieds, or links pages (see Figure 5.4). You can even scan the job board to find the biking-related job of your dreams!

Figure 5.4

Cyber Cyclery provides a Web community for cyclists.

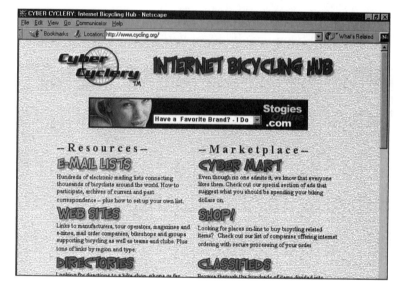

Cardiovascular Machines

Cardiovascular Machine Workouts

    http://primusweb.com/fitnesspartner/library/activity/cardiowork.htm

The Fitness Partner Jumpsite understands that "getting acquainted with the various forms of cardio equipment can be a bit daunting," so they've developed guidelines and 30-minute sample workouts for the treadmill, stationary cycle, stair climber, NordicTrack, and rowing machine.

Walking Magazine's 20 Best Treadmill Workouts

    http://members.aol.com/rayzwocker/worldclass/treadmil.htm

Check out these entertaining walking workouts for those times when Jack Frost is nipping at your nose. "With a little creativity, a treadmill workout can be just as satisfying as an outdoor jaunt."

Aerobic Exercise Classes/Videos

Aerobics at drkoop.com

    http://www.drkoop.com/wellness/fitness/facts/aerobics.asp

This site gives you the full scoop on group exercise classes: advantages, disadvantages, recommended attire, guidelines, and a glossary explaining different types of classes.

Spinning on the Internet

http://www.spinning.com

This is the official resource for Spinning, a group cycling class that's taking the world by storm!

BodyPump

http://www.bodypump.com

Here's the latest info on the group exercise class that combines weight training with an aerobic workout.

Jazzercise

http://www.jazzercise.com

One of the original group exercise classes, Jazzercise is still going strong after 30 years. Search for a class in your area.

Turnstep.com

http://www.turnstep.com

A library of aerobic choreography patterns. Great resource for instructors or if you want to design your own workout at home!

Kickboxing

http://www.afaa.com/

AFAA (The Aerobics and Fitness Association of America) presents tips for enjoying aerobic kickboxing and preventing risk of injury. Find them by clicking **What's Hot** and then **The ABC's of KickBoxing**. Then click **Photos of Correct/Incorrect Form** to learn how to do the boxing stance and various punches and kicks. Clicking Kickboxing Video Training Tips gives technique instruction with little video clips if you have a Java-enabled browser.

Collage Video

http://www.collagevideo.com/

Exercise videos let you work out with top-flight instructors in the privacy of your own home. You can work out at midnight, talk back to the instructor, wear ragged sweats, and pause or fast-forward whenever you please. Collage Video, in business since 1987, has hundreds of workout videos for you to choose from, and most are not available in stores.

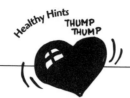

Starting Out in Aerobics Class

Group aerobics classes are a terrific way to get in shape, especially if you enjoy dance and the energy of other people. If you're a newcomer, give yourself several classes to get used to an instructor's style, steps, and cue words. The main purpose of the choreography is to keep you moving, so make that *your* goal, too. When the arms and legs are too confusing, do just the footwork, or march in place and do just the arms. If you get winded, don't push. Take a break for water, or just walk in place. Don't worry if you can't complete the class at first. It gets easier.

It Doesn't Have to Feel Like "Exercise"

We prefer the term "aerobic activity" instead of "exercise" because you can enjoy the benefits of a heart-strengthening workout doing social or leisure activities that you might not even consider exercise. Why not take a ballroom dancing class with your partner? You'll get a great workout and impress your friends and family at the next wedding you attend. Or how about line-dancing or a hike with a friend? How about a favorite sport? For more ideas, read on to Chapter 9, "Recreational Activities: Fun and Fitness."

The Least You Need to Know

➤ Aerobic activity strengthens your heart, helps control weight, reduces stress, and is a necessary part of any fitness program.

➤ Perform aerobic activity at least 30 minutes a day, three days a week at the proper intensity for your fitness level.

➤ "Aerobics" doesn't just mean aerobic dance class—it can be walking, running, rollerblading, swimming, dancing, raking leaves, or just about any rhythmic activity.

➤ You can find information, classes, clubs, and technique for any aerobic activity online.

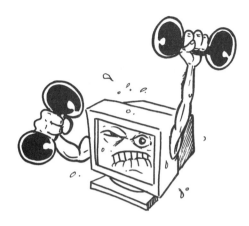

Chapter 6

Strength Training: Not Just for Bodybuilders

In This Chapter

➤ Understanding the basics of strength training

➤ Learning how to achieve your fitness goals with strength training

➤ Finding strength-training programs and information online

Weight loss; injury and disease prevention; and toned, defined muscles are just a few of the rewards of strength training. Working out with weights used to belong in a man's world, but researchers now extol the benefits of strength training for men and women, the young, the old, the slim, and the overweight.

There are *millions* of strength-training related Web sites on the Internet. Sorting out the valuable information from the misinformation is not an easy task, especially when the experts themselves are not always in agreement on the best way to train your body with weights. Although there are different methods of strength training, there are also some time-tested basics, which we outline for you in this chapter. Then we guide you to credible Web sites that offer more detailed information.

Important Reasons Why You Need to Strength Train

Strength training, also known as weight training or resistance training, means exercising with weights or other resistance devices that stress the muscles to the point that they cope by getting stronger. You can lift weights, or push and pull on strength-training machines, or use resistance tools such as Dyna-Bands (see the description in Chapter 11, "Hit the Road: Health and Fitness Resorts, Spas, and Vacations") or rubber tubing. The point is to make the muscles work hard to do the lifting (or pushing or pulling), so that they have to get stronger.

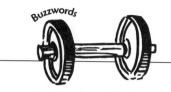

Buzzwords

Strength Training: Working your muscles against resistance so that they have to get stronger.

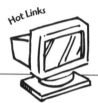

Hot Links

Twelve Reasons Every Adult Should Do Strength Exercise

http://www.healthy.net/library/ articles/westcott/ twelvereasons.htm

This article by strength-training researcher Wayne L. Wescott, Ph.D., presents 12 reasons to work your muscles, and backs up each one with research.

You might be tempted to skip this chapter, especially if you are a woman or a senior. Read on—this is important stuff. Strength training—which used to be relegated to muscle-bound men who grunted and grimaced under heavily loaded barbells—is for *everyone*.

After age 45, women and men lose muscle strength and muscle mass at the rate of five percent per decade, and even faster if they don't exercise at all. By their late 70s, one-third of all men and two-thirds of all women cannot lift an object weighing 10 pounds! That's a sack of cat food! Adding—and preserving—muscle is beneficial for everyone, no matter what your age or gender.

Strength training can

➤ Make you stronger and better able to perform daily life tasks with ease.

➤ Help you lose weight by increasing your metabolism. Muscle burns more calories than fat, even when your body is at rest.

➤ Increase your balance and coordination.

➤ Decrease your risk of osteoporosis and bone breaks, as well as protecting your joints against injury. For example, stronger leg muscles mean less chance of knee injuries.

➤ Keep you strong and independent for decades.

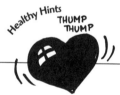

Healthy Hints THUMP THUMP

Lifting Weights Relieves Anxiety

Do you have a stressful meeting coming up in a few hours? A blind date? A visit from your mother? Strength training can relieve your anxiety so you can sail through your stressful event! A report published in *Medicine & Science in Sports & Exercise* demonstrated the surprising results that a single session of moderate-weight resistance training significantly reduced anxiety in male and female study volunteers three hours after training. For the full story, see http:// www.fitnessmotivation.com/articles.htm.

Understanding Strength-Training Basics

If you're a beginner to strength training, or if you've never done it at all, don't be intimidated by the bodybuilding sites (or magazines or TV shows) that show Popeye-muscled men and women. If that's not your aim and you don't spend *many* hours a week pushing yourself to your limits, you won't develop big muscles. With a consistent, moderate program of strength training, you'll get strong, sleek, defined muscles—you won't get big and bulky.

Here's the truth about muscles:

➤ If you don't use 'em, you lose 'em. Muscles don't just stay the same with disuse; they lose strength and, eventually, function.

➤ If you do use 'em right, you can gain strength, function, balance, energy, independence, stronger bones, flexibility, and a trim-and-tight physique—even if you're out of shape when you start working out.

➤ You can make dramatic gains in muscle strength with two sessions a week, but you must use weights or other resistance heavy enough to force the muscles to get stronger. Dozens of repetitions using the lightest weights will minimally improve muscle strength. Soup cans just won't do it. Weights heavy enough to make the muscles react will do it.

➤ It isn't enough to do aerobic exercise. Muscles need site-specific attention. You can run or hike all day long and still lose arm, back, shoulder, and chest strength.

➤ Women: You will not get the female bodybuilder look from strength training; rather, you'll become more shapely. Women who get masculine-looking from strength lifting use monstrously heavy weights, work out many hours a day, diet stringently, have more testosterone (male hormone) than normal, and often take anabolic steroids.

> **Hot Links**
>
> **Can Strength Training Make a Woman Bulky?**
>
> http://ocean.st.usm.edu/ ~mschowal/
>
> This research-paper Web page discusses the health benefits of strength training and why women need not worry about "bulking up."

So, are you convinced? A basic knowledge of how your muscles work helps you achieve your goals. After you have the strength-training habit and you're ready to tweak your program and go beyond the basics, we recommend having a certified personal trainer individualize your program. Here's what you need to understand to get started.

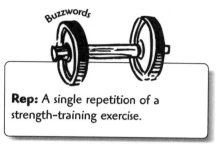

Rep: A single repetition of a strength-training exercise.

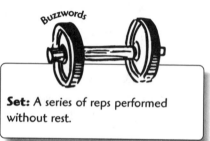

Set: A series of reps performed without rest.

Reps and Sets

Each time you lift and lower a weight, or push and pull against resistance, is called a "repetition," abbreviated "rep." A set is a number of reps done in a row without resting in between. A basic strength-training routine consists of one or two sets of eight to 12 reps of one exercise per muscle group. If you do more than one set, rest for 60 to 90 seconds between sets. Always stretch at the end.

How Much Weight?

When developing a strength-training program, you need to test out different amounts of weight to determine how much you should be lifting. The proper amount of weight enables you to perform eight to 12 repetitions before the muscle becomes fatigued or "fails"—meaning you can't do one more rep with good form. If you can easily perform more than two sets of 12 reps, you should move on to a higher weight. If you can't eke out eight reps, the weight is too heavy.

Too light, and your muscles don't get stronger. Too heavy, and you risk injury. Your muscles are different strengths—your back and thigh muscles are much stronger than your shoulders and arms, for example; so you need heavier weights for your large muscles and lighter ones for the smaller muscles.

How Often?

Rest is just as important as work when it comes to strength training. Muscles become stronger when you've pushed them to their limit and then let them rest for a day to repair. A good guideline to follow is to wait 48 hours between strength-training workouts for the same muscle group—this gives your muscles time to adapt and get stronger.

Triceps Dips

This exercise uses your body weight to strengthen the backs of your upper arms, called the triceps. (You know, the saggy part of your arm that keeps waving after your hand stops!)

1. Sit on the edge of a sturdy chair, hands on the chair on each side of you, fingertips pointing toward your knees. Keeping your weight on your hands, push your buttocks off the chair and walk your feet out until your buttocks are "sitting" on air, and your body weight is supported by your hands on the chair.

2. Slowly bend your elbows, lowering your buttocks part-way down toward the floor. If you're strong enough, bend until your elbows make a 90-degree angle. If not, just go to where you feel the difficulty.

3. Straighten your arms (without locking your elbows), pushing your body weight back up. Repeat the motion slowly as many times as you can. (If this is easy, walk your feet farther away to put more weight on your arms.)

4. Watch yourself in a mirror or have someone else check your form. Be careful that you're not just dipping your body without bending your arms—your arms must bend and straighten to work these muscles.

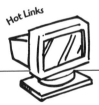

Strong Women Stay Young and *Strong Women Stay Slim*

http://www.strongwomen.com

These two ground-breaking books by Tufts researcher Miriam E. Nelson, Ph.D., and Sarah Wernick became best sellers, teaching women the value of strength training and giving them simple, effective programs to follow with a minimum of equipment. Click **Free Newsletter** to sign up for a monthly e-letter with strength-training tips, Q & A from readers, and healthy recipes.

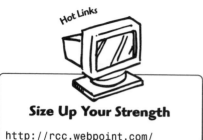

Hot Links

Size Up Your Strength

http://rcc.webpoint.com/
fitness/strength.htm

How strong are you? Take this three-part strength-assessment test; no equipment necessary.

Getting the Results You Want

There are different ways to strength train and not one of them is right for everyone. Your best bet is to educate yourself and always keep your personal goals in mind. Seeing results depends on training properly. You don't need a bodybuilder's workout if your goal is to tone your muscles and maintain strength. Likewise, a workout with lighter weights and higher repetitions will not give you the physique of Schwarzenegger.

If your aim is to get stronger but not become a bodybuilder, a consistent program of strength training the basic muscles with one or two sets each, two to three days a week on nonconsecutive days, will do it. As soon as your weights feel easier and you can do more than 12 repetitions, increase the weight.

As much as you hate to hear this, we have to clear up one common myth: There's no such thing as spot reducing. Under no circumstances can you make a specific part of your body smaller with a resistance exercise! Sorry! Leg lifts do not make your thighs smaller. Crunches do not make your stomach flat. As we discussed in Chapter 5, "Aerobics: Raising Your Heart Rate Online," aerobic activity is the only way to reduce body fat and get "smaller." Strength training or "toning" exercises can give your muscles shapely definition, but those muscles won't show if there is a layer of fat on top of them. Every exercise regimen should include aerobic activity to complement strength training.

Start Here: Basic Strength-Training Sites

These sites will help you begin a strength-training program, even if you've never lifted weights before.

The Complete Guide to Strength Training

http://www.fitnesslink.com/exercise/guide.htm

This site is a complete how-to guide for strength training for the beginner to the bodybuilder. How to begin a strength training program, what equipment you need, and a complete list of exercises for every muscle group.

Fitness Online

http://www.fitnessonline.com

This site uses content from the Weider magazines—*Shape, Flex, Muscle & Fitness, Men's Fitness, Natural Health,* and *Fit Pregnancy* (see Figure 6.1). Click **Exercise**, and then **Strength Training** for a selection of articles from these magazines.

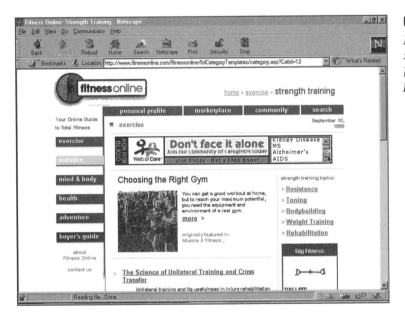

Figure 6.1

Fitness Online offers strength-training articles from popular Weider publications.

Strength Training

http://www.gsu.edu/~wwwfit/strength.html

Georgia State University tells you how to get started, describes strength-training principles, and gives you a sample strength-training program.

Training for Strength

http://www.ama-assn.org/insight/gen_hlth/trainer/strength.htm

This site, from the American Medical Association, gives you the basics about why and how to strength train, including guidelines from the American College of Sports Medicine and nine simple, beginning-level, illustrated exercises.

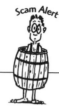

Scam Alert

"Expert" Advice: Use Caution

We came across a Web site whose introduction stated, "Welcome to my attempt at a comprehensive weight training course." It would be nice if all sites were as honest about their content. But in reality, there are many people who publish Web sites on strength training, claiming to be "experts" or to have "the most effective" programs. Always remember to use the PILOT method when evaluating a Web site, and pay special attention to the "Originator." If the site doesn't state the credentials of the person giving out the advice, you would be wise to seek out a more credible site.

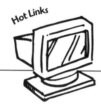

Hot Links

Tools to Help You Develop Your Strength-Training Workout

The following Web sites are valuable resources when putting together your strength-training workout. Use these sites to learn more about muscles and exercises, or to add life to a stale program.

ExRx Online http://www.planetkc.com/exrx/Exercise.html
Whether you're looking for strength-training exercises to add to your routine or a deeper understanding of how your muscles work, this site offers nearly 300 animated exercise demos with complete descriptions of the muscles involved.

Global Health & Fitness http://www.global-fitness.com/strength.html
Click **Muscle Map** to find a photograph with muscles labeled. When you click a muscle, you get a description of the muscle and exercises that work it.

Jean-Paul Fitness Specialists http://www.jeanpaul.com/workouts.html
This site includes six different strength-training programs, complete with photo demonstrations, as well as solid advice on strength training for the strength-training athlete who needs to pep up his or her program.

Bodybuilding

Most men and some women are not content with getting stronger for health—they want bigger muscles. Increasing muscle mass requires training with heavier weights and committing to a longer strength-training workout. Bodybuilders usually work out most days of the week, doing a split routine, which means they work certain muscles one day and different muscles the next. That way, they give individual muscles the rest days we talked about, but still work out almost every day. They also do several different exercises and multiple sets for each muscle group.

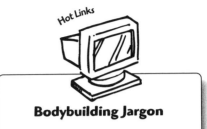

Bodybuilding Jargon

http://www.getbig.com/
glossary/jargon.htm

Bodybuilding has its own language. American Bodybuilding defines some common terms.

Start Here: Bodybuilding Sites

There are a number of different training philosophies and techniques, and you can find them all on the Web. With the overwhelming amount of strength training and bodybuilding information online, it's tough to sort it all out. To help you get a start, we've done some extensive searching and the following sites get "two biceps up."

American Bodybuilding

> http://www.getbig.com

If you're into competitive bodybuilding—doing it or watching it—this site has body building info galore: contest results, competition information, articles, photos, magazines, nutrition products, links, chat, and bulletin boards.

Bill Pearl

> http://www.billpearl.com/ (click on "programs")

Bill Pearl, winner of many top bodybuilding titles, provides complete bodybuilding workouts with photo demonstrations in "20 Months to a Champion Physique."

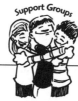

Strength-Training Support

The Internet is a great place to ask questions and get advice on strength training and bodybuilding. Check out the following interactive resources:

➤ `misc.fitness.weights` A newsgroup devoted to strength-training issues.

➤ `http://www.getbig.com/board2/board2.cgi` A Q & A bulletin board at American Bodybuilding.

➤ `http://www.weightsnet.com/weights/` Weights mailing list.

➤ `http://www.muscle-fitness.com` Muscle & Fitness Magazine Online has live chats with fitness celebrities and an active bulletin board.

➤ `http://staff.washington.edu/griffin/weights.html` Weighty Matters is an archive of selected posts from various strength-training newsgroups, mailing lists, and chats.

CyberPump

`http://www.cyberpump.com`

This is a fun site with lots to offer the strength-training or bodybuilding enthusiast. Spend some time surfing through the "features" section for "information on various aspects of the weight game." Learn about H.I.T.—High Intensity Training ("going all out, not almost all out...taking one set to one's absolute limit")—at `http://www.cyberpump.com/hitfaq/`.

Periodization of Strength

`http://sa.acusd.edu/users/WeightRoom/periodiz.html`

Periodization is the process of structuring training into phases that vary through the year or training cycle. Learn about it in this article from the University of San Diego.

Testosterone: "Muscle with Attitude"

`http://www.testosterone.net`

Everything you could ever want to know about building muscle is in this spunky online magazine, written in a jaunty, renegade, man-to-man style. Get training routines and tips from strength guru Charles Poliquin.

The Least You Need to Know

➤ Strength training is an important part of every fitness program—no matter what your age or gender.

➤ Learning to train properly helps you achieve your desired results.

➤ The Internet is chock-full of strength-training information and misinformation; use the PILOT method and remember to keep your goals in mind when considering any workout program.

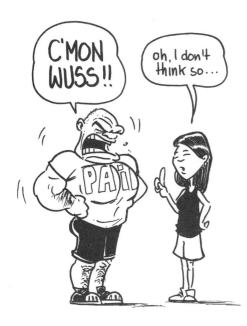

Chapter 7

Personal Trainers: Finding One That's Right for You

In This Chapter

➤ Using a personal trainer to help you achieve your fitness goals

➤ Finding a personal trainer that's right for you

➤ Locating a personal trainer using online resources

A personal trainer is your coach, motivator, and teacher. Whether you're a beginning exerciser or a seasoned athlete, a personal trainer can provide motivation, fitness education, exercise instruction, fitness testing, program design, and goal assessment. Your trainer applauds your progress and eases you through the tough spots. If you've never worked with a personal trainer, we recommend trying it once—you might just get hooked!

Working with a personal trainer also adds accountability: You've paid good money to work with your trainer, so you'd better show up for your scheduled appointments and work as hard as you can!

Where do our online tools come into play when finding a personal trainer? The Web offers personal trainer directories, articles on finding a trainer, motivational articles and advice written by trainers, and even trainers who will "train" you via email.

What Does a Trainer Do?

A good trainer sits down with you and talks to you about your goals, your exercise preferences, your history, any medical considerations, and your barriers. With his or her help, you'll think about exercise options that you would enjoy doing—not just activities where you have to grit your teeth and count the minutes. For example, you might think you have to get on that boring stair climber and climb to nowhere for 30 minutes. But your personal trainer might suggest a more appealing activity that gives you the same or better workout.

Your trainer will test your fitness level—which we discussed in Chapter 4, "Developing Your Personal Fitness Program,"—and help you design a workout that you can stick to. So many of us work out with an exercise video, or lift some weights at the gym, and never see the results we hope for because we're not doing the right type of workout to achieve our goals. Your personal trainer shows you what exercises to do, how to perform them correctly, and inspires you to stick with it—especially if you are paying your trainer week after week to work out with you!

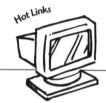

Hot Links

Is Personal Training for You?

http://www.ideafit.com/ftptforyou.cfm

This article from IDEA, The Health and Fitness Source, details what a trainer does and how you can tell whether you'd benefit from working with one. It's written by Larry Dyke, MS, director of personal training for the Australian Body Works, a 15-club chain in Atlanta, Georgia.

Do You Need a Trainer? The Pros and Cons

There are many, many "pros" to working out with a personal trainer. After you make your first appointment, you'll see how empowering it can be. A personal trainer can help you to see new ways to exercise, stay motivated, and take control of achieving your goals. The personal relationship itself often helps you stick with it—you know another person is charting your progress and cares whether you show up.

We can't think of many "cons" against working with a personal trainer—other than the financial commitment—but you do need to be sure you find the right one for you. A trainer who isn't well-educated, doesn't have your best interests in mind, or doesn't match your personality can have a detrimental effect on your training program.

Pushups

What would a chapter on personal trainers be without pushups? Whether you do pushups with bent or straight legs, be sure to keep your head, neck, and spine in line (don't drop your head or let your back arch) and the abdominals contracted through the whole sequence. Lower by bending your arms (not by sagging your belly!) and raise your body by straightening your arms. On the way down, let your chest lead—don't dip the chin or forehead. Go slowly: no faster than 2 seconds down and 2 seconds up, and go even slower if you're strong. Exhale on the way up. This is the most effective all-purpose upper-body strengthener—it's well worth the effort!

What to Look For: Finding a Trainer Online and Off

Whether you're searching for your personal trainer on the Internet or through your local health club, physician, or Yellow Pages, use the following criteria to find one that's right for you.

Education

You will rely on your trainer to provide you with the latest fitness information. Does your trainer keep current by attending fitness education events, taking college courses, and reading trade publications? Does she or he know the exercise recommendations for people of your age or with your medical condition?

Certification

Your should have a degree in an exercise physiology, medical, or physical science field or hold a certification through a nationally recognized organization. FitnessLink offers a list of certification organizations at http://www.fitnesslink.com/fitpro/proassoc.htm. Your trainer should be certified in CPR and first aid.

Experience

Does the trainer have experience with people like you? Can he or she provide references from satisfied clients and/or medical professionals? Your trainer should be experienced in fitness assessment, goal-setting, and training instruction.

Individualization

If a trainer has a set program he or she teaches every client, despite personal goals or challenges, look for another trainer. If you're 60 years old, you won't do the same workout as a 30-year-old. If you have arthritis, carpal tunnel syndrome, a bad back, or any other medical condition that can be worsened by the wrong kind of exercise, you want a trainer who knows how to give you a program that helps without hurting.

Professionalism

Does the trainer arrive on time for appointments, and concentrate fully on you while you're together? Your trainer is not there to get his or her own workout, but to assist you. Your trainer's dress should be appropriate (some of us don't feel inspired by ragged sweats) and not intimidating (some of us would rather not view the trainer's belly-button ring).

Policies

Your trainer should provide you with clear policies on cancellations and billing, preferably in writing. A trainer should also be able to explain his or her workout methods (this might also be in writing) and the reasoning behind them.

Liability Insurance

Your trainer should carry professional liability insurance in case you get injured.

Fees

Is the trainer's fee within your budget? Trainers charge a wide range of fees depending on location and the trainer's experience and reputation. A trainer who is greatly in demand commands a higher fee than one who is looking for clients. This person might or might not be better for you than a beginner trying to establish a clientele—so shop around, and interview prospective trainers.

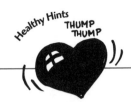

Keep the "Personal" in Personal Trainer

A woman phoned Joan and said, "I understand you're good with out-of-shape beginners. A friend and I want to start working with a personal trainer. Tell me what you would do with us."

Joan said, "I can't tell you that until I learn more about you. Talk to me about who you are, your goals, your lifestyle, your exercise history, and your challenges."

The caller said, "You're hired. Every other trainer we called launched into an explanation of her perfect workout program. You're the only one who wanted to know more about us first."

The moral of the story is this: A personal trainer must be committed to personalizing your program so that you'll get what *you* need to succeed.

Personality

You need to feel comfortable with and motivated by your trainer. Does she or he listen and communicate well with you? Look at what type of personality suits you best: A drill sergeant? A cheerleader? An educator? An entertainer? A gentle handholder? Do you prefer to work with a man or woman?

If you plan to use your trainer as a consultant—to develop your program initially, and then meet with occasionally for a progress check—personality isn't as important as expertise. But if you want to use your trainer as a partner—to motivate your workouts on a regular basis—personality is crucial. Look for someone you'll look forward to seeing on a regular basis.

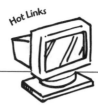

Hot Links

Trainers Answer Your Questions

Several trainers have posted answers to frequently asked questions (FAQs) on their Web sites. Here are a couple of respected trainers who offer solid advice about exercise, weight loss, and related topics that might be on your mind:

➤ **Personal trainer Greg Niederlander**
http://www.ring.com/health/ptrainer.htm

➤ **Personal trainer Jack Dixon**   http://lifematters.com/jackfaq.html

Personal Training via Email: Serious Scam Potential

You might get lucky and find a personal trainer hanging out in a fitness chat rooms offering dandy, free advice about training principles and motivation. This can pep up your program and encourage you to get started, keep going, or try something new. You can also read some inspiring articles and get your basic questions answered online by a professional trainer. But what about trainers who, for a fee, train you online?

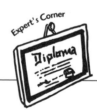

Expert's Corner

Diploma

"I've given training advice in online chats. There are some principles that people don't understand that are easily explainable online. For example, a guy says he's been doing barbell curls for six months and his biceps stopped getting bigger after the second month. So, it's pretty easy to explain to that guy that he needs to try different exercises, different sets and reps, and so on, to start getting results again. I don't have to measure his blood pressure and take a health history to give him that advice."

—Lou Schuler, certified personal trainer, fitness editor of *Men's Health* magazine

When you search the Web for personal trainers, you will find many that offer "online" training services. This can be anything from general fitness advice (see Figure 7.1) to a complete assessment and program design. Some provide you with a detailed fitness program, help you track your workouts and progress, and even email you motivational reminders each day!

Online training can work for those who cannot or will not go to a gym, who can't afford a trainer in their area, or who might be embarrassed to exercise in front of someone else. But there are serious drawbacks you need to realize. The idea behind "personal" training is meeting with someone face-to-face who can personally evaluate your particular needs and goals. A personal trainer is there to demonstrate proper technique and evaluate yours. He or she spots you when you lift weights.

With online training, you don't get these benefits. There isn't a live person there to hold you accountable when you skip a day of training. The trainer is not there to check your form or protect you from doing an exercise incorrectly. The trainer might not be experienced or educated (you can't believe everything you read on the Web!), might not care enough to develop a program that's going to help you reach your goals (you might get a "template" workout—the same workout he or she gives to everyone else!), or might not deliver what you pay for at all.

If you do decide to use an online trainer, be sure you know what you are paying for. Evaluate the trainer's site using the PILOT method. Check references carefully. Verify credentials. Find out how long the trainer has been operating online so you won't be left with a disappearing act after you give your credit card number.

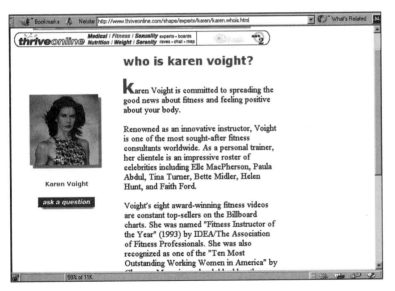

Figure 7.1

Karen Voight, fitness authority and personal trainer to the stars, answers your questions at Thrive Online, `http://thriveonline. com/shape/experts /karen/karen.today. html`.

Start Here: Searching for Personal Trainers Online

American Council on Exercise

```
http://www.acefitness.org/profreg/
```

ACE is one of the major certifying organizations for group-exercise leaders and personal trainers. You can search by region for ACE-certified trainers. Clicking a name gives you more information, including education, specialties, phone number, fee, and preferred types of clients.

Total Fitness Guide

```
http://totalfitnessguide.com
```

Search online for a trainer in your area, or email the site for a recommendation.

Health and Fitness Network

```
http://www.healthfitnessnetwork.com
```

Click "Trainer/Gym Locator" to search for a trainer in your area.

The Least You Need to Know

➤ Personal trainers can show you how to develop a fitness program that meets your needs and helps you achieve your goals.

➤ When searching for a trainer, consider his or her certification, experience, professionalism, references, fees, insurance, and personality.

➤ The Internet can be useful in helping you search for a trainer in your area, but be cautious when using "online" trainers.

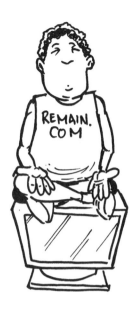

Chapter 8

Mind/Body Fitness: Stretching, Yoga, Martial Arts, and More

In This Chapter

➤ Adding awareness to your fitness regimen

➤ Using mind/body techniques to enhance the quality of your workouts and help you achieve your goals

➤ Choosing a mind/body fitness activity using the Internet

The "no-pain, no-gain" fitness class of the '80s has given way to a more mindful generation of workouts called "mind/body" exercise. Mind/body workouts—such as yoga, Pilates, stretching, and martial arts—encourage you to put your mind where your muscle is. By increasing your awareness of muscle work, breathing, and joint movement, as well as incorporating positive affirmations and goals into your workouts, you can improve your fitness performance and move closer to your goals.

This chapter guides you through a journey into mind/body exercises using the World Wide Web as a pathway.

Adding Awareness to Your Workout: The Mind/Body Connection

In our rushed, hectic lives, we're often stressed from the minute we're awakened by the buzz of the alarm clock to the minute we fall asleep late at night, often with the

TV news still blaring. If we exercise at all, we tend to compartmentalize it—rush to the gym or jogging route, work out with one eye on our watch, rush to shower, and take on the day.

Stop. Close your eyes. Take several deep breaths. Visualize yourself looking healthy, fit, and relaxed. Repeat a verbal affirmation: "I feel strong, calm, and in peak condition."

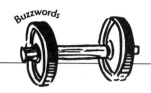

Mind/Body: Exercise technique that incorporates deep breathing, mental focus and visualization to result in stress reduction, motivation, and enhanced physical performance.

Incorporating relaxation techniques, mind/body awareness, and affirmations into your daily routine helps you enjoy your life with less stress. Including them within your workouts heightens the results— you can accomplish more, because your mind is assisting.

Athletes, celebrities, busy executives, and ordinary folks are all discovering the benefits of exercising with the mind involved as well as the body. In addition to increasing your fitness performance and helping you stay motivated, mind/body techniques can help you reduce stress, and take a more balanced approach to life's challenges.

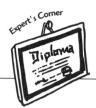

"People think that mind/body methods are mysterious and complicated, when they are really just the opposite. Mind/body simply means that your mind and body are working together, focusing on the same thing at the same time. It's about self-awareness...paying attention in every moment and putting your whole self into everything you do."

—Gloria Keeling, founder of Strong, Stretched & Centered Mind-Body Fitness Training Institute, http://www.mauifitness.com

Mind/Body Exercise for a Fit, Healthy Body

When it comes to exercise and sports performance, mind/body means truly experiencing your workout, focusing on your performance and/or your goals, reveling in the benefits your body is enjoying, and visualizing yourself achieving your goals. Instead of reading a magazine or staring at the television during your workout, try one of these techniques:

➤ Look at your workout as something to be enjoyed, not endured. That hour that you spend exercising is *your* time—time to be alone, to think, to relax, and to appreciate the good things you are doing for your body and mind. During your workout, the only responsibility you have is to yourself and the healthy body you are building.

➤ When cycling, imagine you are racing in the Tour de France and you're in the lead. See the nearest competitor riding on your heels, about to overtake you. Put in that extra effort to stay ahead and win the race. This technique also works well if you are training for a marathon or any other racing event.

➤ Visualize your muscles as you work out. See them contracting, stretching, and growing stronger. Concentrating on a specific muscle group helps you to work that muscle harder, and it responds more intensely.

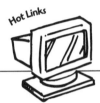

Hot Links

Brain Workouts for a Better Body

http://www.fitnesslink.com/mind/brainwrk.htm

Want a sure-fire performance enhancer? Faster progress, more results? Researchers are now proving what the winners always knew: Put your mental power behind your muscles, and get ready for big-time results. Joan shows you how in this article.

Using the Web to Make the Connection

Now that you understand what mind/body means, you can turn to the Internet for information on mind/body fitness techniques and ways you can incorporate self-awareness into your workouts.

Stretching

Are you one of those people who forgets to stretch, or doesn't think it's worth the time? Do you figure it's just for the weak or injured? Flexibility is one of the major components of fitness, yet stretching is the most neglected element in most fitness routines. Stretching is essential for preventing injury and improving range of motion and performance.

Stretching is an effective mind/body technique. You tune into how your body feels and how the relaxation of stretching releases stress. You become aware of which muscles are tight and how you can use your stretch to lengthen them.

Before you begin your stretch, inhale deeply. Then sink into the stretch, exhaling slowly. When you reach the point of a comfortable stretch, breathe normally, and on each exhalation, sink a little bit deeper into the stretch. Concentrate on the muscle you are stretching, feeling it become loose and relaxed. Never force a stretch or bounce.

Phys.com's "Reach for Your Health," `http://www.phys.com/f_fitness/02solutions/03stretching/stretching.html`, offers an informative list of stretching do's and don'ts as well as a complete, illustrated stretching routine (see Figure 8.1).

Figure 8.1

PHYS gives you the low-down on stretching.

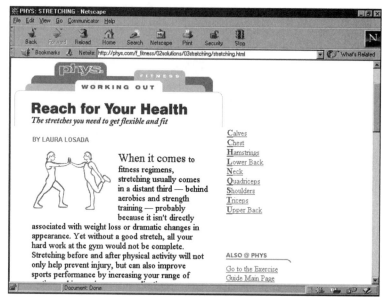

Online Stretches

Go to `http://www.shelterpub.com` and click **Online Stretches**. This takes you to a page from Bob Anderson's *Stretching at Your Computer or Desk*, with eight illustrated stretches for you to do *right now* for your tense shoulders and neck and overworked wrists. (Go ahead. We'll wait.)

Yoga is thousands of years old, and is being discovered anew by more than six million American exercisers, who find it a powerful stress-reduction tool and an antidote to their frenetic lifestyle. Although yoga has its roots in ancient Indian philosophy, today it has become a popular method of mind/body fitness, incorporating flexibility, muscle strength, balance, coordination, stress reduction, and mental clarity. There are many different types of yoga classes, ranging from slow, peaceful poses to "power yoga" which offers mental focus as well as an intense aerobic workout.

To learn more about yoga online, get started with the following sites.

Yoga Site

```
http://www.yogasite.com
```

In addition to the Yoga FAQ, the posture page, and the links to yoga Web sites, organizations, newsgroups, mailing lists, and publications, you'll find a teacher directory where you can search your state for a yoga instructor near you.

Sivananda Yoga "Om" Page

```
http://www.sivananda.org/
```

More than 300 pages, 450 graphics, plus audio clips and animated illustrations immerse you in yoga. This is the official site of the International Sivananda Yoga Vedanta Centers, committed to "teaching Yoga authentically, preserving its purity and tradition." Read the principles of yoga, and then look at photos and descriptions of basic and advanced asanas (postures). This site even has "spiritual jokes."

Part 1: What did the Yogi say when he walked into the Zen Pizza Parlor? "Make me one with everything."

Part 2: When the Yogi got the pizza, he gave the proprietor a $20 bill. The proprietor pocketed the bill. The Yogi asked, "Don't I get change?" The proprietor said, "Change must come from within."

YOGAaahhh Asanas

```
http://www2.gdi.net/~mjm/asana.html
```

The YOGAaahhh Web site presents 30 hatha yoga poses with complete descriptions and illustrations (see Figure 8.2).

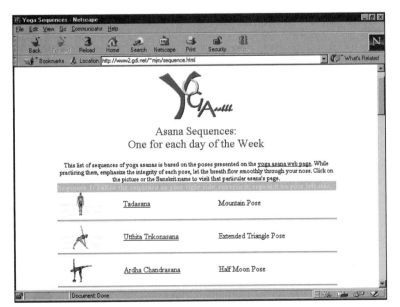

Figure 8.2

Get a complete sequence of yoga poses from the YOGAaahhh Web site.

Pilates

Pilates originated as rehabilitation for injured soldiers during World War I and developed into rehabilitation and conditioning for dancers. Now, everyday exercisers have discovered the benefits of improved posture, breathing, concentration, flexibility, endurance, and coordination, and an overall longer, leaner body.

Pilates has been described as a combination of calisthenics and yoga. The exercises, which stretch the muscles and strengthen the "core" of the body (the torso and hip area), are performed on special, spring-loaded apparatus. There is also a form of Pilates, known as "matwork," that can be done without any equipment.

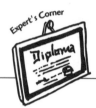

"Mind/body exercise is not necessarily about 'what' you do, but 'how' you do it. When you focus the mind on how the body moves, you are able to develop strength, balance, and flexibility while eliminating stress."

—Moira Stott, Program Director, STOTT Pilates Studios & International Certification Center, `http://www.stottconditioning.com`

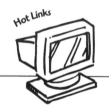

How to Choose a Pilates Instructor

`http://www.stottconditioning.com/NR07_howchse.html`

Stott Conditioning details 10 key questions to ask your Pilates instructor, raising issues such as certification, benefits, and equipment.

Pilates: Matwork, Exercises, and Equipment

`http://www.bodymind.net`

Visit this site for a list of Pilates studios and instructors worldwide, as well as videos, books, frequently asked questions, links, and a mailing list.

The Pilates Studio

`http://www.pilates-studio.com`

Click **The Method** to read about what Pilates is and how you can benefit from it.

Martial Arts

Judo, Karate, Aikido, Jujutsu, and Tai Chi are just a few of the martial arts. Originally, all the martial arts were fighting forms, as the name indicates. Over the centuries, some—Tai Chi is a prime example—have evolved into gentle, graceful exercise traditions that seem far removed from fighting. Others are still forms of combat, frequently taught as self-defense.

Because there are so many martial arts, exploring them all online would become a book in itself. To get started, here are some helpful sites.

WWW Martial Arts Resource Page

http://www.middlebury.edu/~jswan/martial.arts/ma.html

This link-rich site is maintained by Middlebury, VT instructor Jay Swan. Read about how to choose a martial arts school, and get links to schools and informational sites to explore dozens of different martial arts.

AikiWeb

http://www.aikiweb.com

Immerse yourself in information about Aikido, a Japanese martial art that focuses on using the opponent's energy to gain control or to deflect an attack (see Figure 8.3). For more, see also Aikido FAQs (http://www.aikidofaq.com).

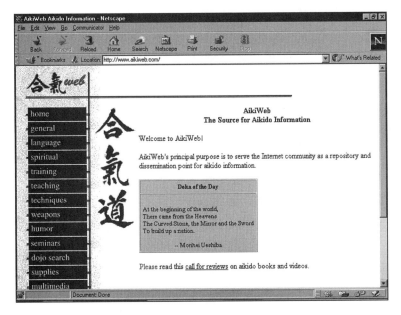

Figure 8.3

AikiWeb is a powerhouse of information on Aikido.

Jujutsu Links

`http://www.middlebury.edu/~jswan/martial.arts/pages/jujutsu.html`

Jujutsu is over 3,000 years old. At the turn of the century, the Japanese government catalogued more than 450 different varieties. There are so many forms (and spellings) of Jujutsu that your best bet is to explore an assortment and decide which appeals to you enough to pursue. This page gives links to a variety of forms from several countries.

Jane Golden's Tai Chi and Qigong

`http://www.goldenjane.com/taiintro.htm`

"The principle of Tai Chi is harmony, not only with outer forces, but within oneself, harmonizing the physical, mental and spiritual aspects of life," says Northern California Tai Chi instructor Jane Golden. Tai Chi, an ancient Chinese martial art, is a flowing series of postures emphasizing grace, balance, agility, and focus.

Judo Information Site

`http://www.rain.org/~ssa/judo.htm`

Judo, a Japanese fighting system, uses throwing, grappling, and choking techniques (taught safely, of course). This site has illustrations (drawings, animations, and photographs) of dozens of Judo techniques.

Sports Psychology

Whether you're a competitive athlete, a weekend warrior, or a member of your company softball team, you can use mind/body techniques to enhance your sports performance.

The Mind Tools: Sport Psychology Web page (`http://www.mindtools.com/page11.html`) offers an inspiring series of articles detailing how to use your mind to control your body and achieve optimal sports performance, and can also be applied to any fitness goal. Topics include goal setting, imagery, and concentration.

The Least You Need to Know

➤ You can learn exercise methods that increase awareness of your body and help to relax your mind.

➤ Yoga, Pilates, martial arts, and stretching are all valuable mind/body disciplines that can help you reduce stress and increase your fitness performance.

➤ The Web can be your teacher as you learn mind/body fitness techniques.

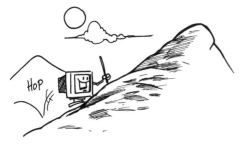

Chapter 9

Recreational Activities: Fun and Fitness

> ### In This Chapter
>
> ➤ Finding ways to make fitness fun
>
> ➤ Using the Web to research and plan outdoor fitness activities
>
> ➤ Dancing as aerobic exercise
>
> ➤ Making fitness a family affair

If the gym is not your destination of choice when you have a free hour, don't fret about it. You can get and stay fit by having fun—if you choose physically energetic recreation. So, instead of renting a video in the evening, go out dancing. Instead of spending a weekend afternoon watching sports on TV, participate in a sport. And for the health and camaraderie of the whole family, take the kids out hiking, biking, or skating. Social and outdoor physical activities are super ways to build active recreation into your week for fitness and stress reduction. This chapter shows you how to use online resources for planning recreational activities that "count" as exercise. Enjoy!

Using the Web to Plan Outdoor Fitness Activities

Incorporating exercise into your daily routine doesn't have to mean suffering through a boring workout program that you don't enjoy. Although some people thrive on treadmill workouts and group exercise classes, they aren't for everyone. You can get an equally effective workout with recreational activities such as biking, skiing, backpacking, and hiking. To plan your next outdoor fitness activity, start with one of these sites:

GORP: The Great Outdoor Recreation Pages

`http://www.gorp.com`

GORP is an outdoor enthusiast's dream—full of articles on tons of outdoor activities from cycling through Italy and kayaking in Alaska to introducing kids to rock climbing. Locate and learn about parks, beaches, rivers, trails, forests, wildlife, recreation, and wilderness areas worldwide. Useful features such as maps, travel, gear, jobs, and forums round out this site (see Figure 9.1).

Figure 9.1

The Great Outdoor Recreation Pages are filled with activity ideas.

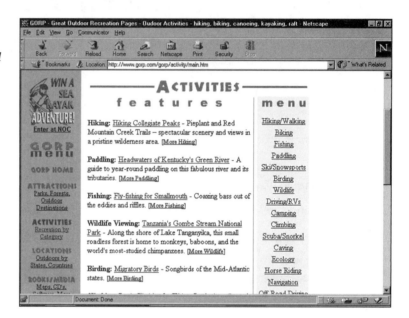

L.L. Bean's Park Search

`http://www.llbean.com`

Just click **Outdoors**, and then **Park Search** to search for a location or activity that interests you, and outdoor products superstore L.L. Bean finds the perfect park for your outdoor fitness adventure. This page includes complete details for more than 1,500 recreation areas in the U.S.—address, phone, fees, activities available, description of the park, and dates each is open.

Outdoor Explorer

`http://www.outdoorexplorer.com`

Whether you camp, hike, bike, paddle, climb, or ski, Outdoor Explorer offers motivating articles, gear reviews, travel information, and weather forecasts. You can look through the personal profiles to find someone in your area who enjoys the same recreational activities as you do. They've also got forums and chat.

Recreation at About.com

    http://home.about.com/sports/recreation/index.htm

Links, articles, forums, and chat on more than 35 recreational activities including golf, canoeing, backpacking, rock climbing, and rowing. Each activity brings up a world of information: techniques, camps, advice, news, and links to dozens of sites. Whether you have a favorite activity and want to learn more about it, or are looking for a new one, you'll find what you seek here.

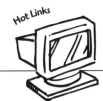

PHYS: Snack Bandit

    http://www.phys.com/c_tools/gadgets/snackbandit/snackbandit.html

How long do you have to brush your teeth to work off a brownie? Try 2 hours and 18 minutes! The Snack Bandit is a fun way to find out just what you have to do to burn off those high-calorie indulgences. Remember that mopping the floor, rearranging furniture, and weeding the garden all count as exercise.

Locating Clubs and Organizations Online

If you enjoy hiking, camping, or any other outdoor activity, but you don't have any pals who share your passion, try joining an organization that puts you in touch with like-minded outdoor fitness enthusiasts. Here are a few places to start surfing:

The Appalachian Long Distance Hikers Association

    http://www.aldha.org/links.htm

This site includes links and info on backpacking and hiking some of America's greatest trails: the Appalachian, the Pacific Crest, and the Continental Divide.

International Mountain Biking Association

    http://www.greatoutdoors.com/imba/

IMBA offers a library of mountain biking articles, a calendar of events, and tips for building and maintaining trails. Check out the "contacts" area (or go directly to `http://www.greatoutdoors.com/imba/contacts/nearyou/clubs.html`) to locate a mountain biking group in your area.

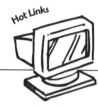

BackWoods Grocery

`http://www.backwoodsgrocery.com`

"Changing the way hikers eat" is an understatement. Shannon used to think that sticking an aluminum foil-wrapped potato in the fire for a half hour was elegant dining on a camping trip, but this site showed her how to really live it up! Start with the campfire cooking primer; then roam their "aisles" to shop for foods you never knew you could enjoy in the great outdoors.

CampUSA

`http://www.campusa.com`

Complete details for thousands of campgrounds across the U.S. Search for a campground by city and/or state, then check out the links section for camping-related sites on the Web.

SkiCentral

`http://www.skicentral.com`

SkiCentral is a must-see site for skiers and snowboarders. This huge jump site provides links to equipment, technique, racing, organization and discussion group Web sites, in addition to resort information, ski reports, and trip planning.

Sierra Club

`http://www.sierraclub.org/`

This environmental organization aims to "explore, enjoy, and protect the wild places of the Earth" through lobbying and campaign support as well as outings and social interaction. Read about hot environmental topics, locate your regional chapter, and join them for a hike or bike ride in your area.

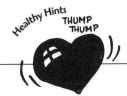

Outdoor Exercise Caution

Each summer, more than 9 million Americans visit the emergency room for ailments such as heatstroke, food poisoning, and exposure to poison ivy. Always carry lots of water and keep picnic and camping foods properly chilled in a cooler. Protect your skin against sun and rash-producing plants by liberally applying sunscreen and a poison ivy "blocking" lotion. Be prepared for cuts and scrapes by bringing along a small first-aid kit containing cotton pads, antiseptic spray or ointment, bandages of various sizes, gauze, and tape.

Get Up and Dance

If you like to dance, you'll love how easy it is to get your aerobic exercise. We've talked about aerobic dance in health clubs in Chapter 5, "Aerobics: Raising Your Heart Rate Online,"—and that's a super way to work out. But social dancing is a way you can get your exercise, enjoy a date with your honey (or, if you're honey-less, meet other singles who love to dance!), and enjoy a social activity that keeps you in shape.

But Is It Exercise?

Is dancing really aerobic? Not if you sit out every other song, or if you concentrate on slow dances such as the waltz. But if you get on the floor and stay there, and your dancing

Dance!

First go to http://www.mrznet. com/smile2.html. While you're waiting for the many dancing graphics to load, warm up by moving to the disco music you hear; then join the dancing raisins, macaroni, dudes, party animals, and babies in some variation of their moves.

gets you breathing faster (and we don't mean because your partner takes your breath away), then, yes, this is aerobic. Some of the best dances for getting your heart rate up and keeping it up are swing (all types, including West Coast swing, East Coast swing, jitterbug, and lindy), country two-step, polka, folk dancing, Cajun, and the fast Latin dances such as salsa. And don't forget good old rock and roll!

Social Dancing

You can find everything dance-oriented, from classes to choreography, on the World Wide Web. Do a search on the kind of dance that interests you, and sort out your results from there. For example, a search on "swing dancing" brought forth these gems along with many other interesting sites:

Archives of Early Lindy Hop

```
http://www.savoystyle.com
```

This site documents the Lindy Hop as it developed at the Savoy in Harlem. It was the precursor to all swing dances, and this site has history, biographies of early swing dancers, Lindy Hop art, movies that featured this dance, and dozens of links. This site comes to you from the SavoyStyle Swing Dance Shop, which sells clothing, videos, and anything related to the Lindy Hop.

Any Swing Goes

```
http://www.anyswinggoes.com
```

This site is a "swing music, news, and culture" online magazine focusing on the revival of big band and swing music and dancing. Read news about your favorite swing bands, and features on how to tie a classic tie (hey, you've gotta dress right!) and swing dance at your wedding.

The US Swing Dance Server

```
http://www.swingcraze.com/ussds/swing_dancing.html
```

This comprehensive site covers all kinds of swing dancing, including places to dance (by type and region), styles, technique, steps, terms, choreography, and links. West Coast swing dancers will appreciate the detailed article, "What Is West Coast Swing?"

Dance Classes

"But I don't know how to dance!" you wail. Again, the Internet comes to the rescue. No, your computer won't dance with you, but you can locate live classes. Whether you want ballroom, country western, folk, swing, tap, ballet, jazz dance, hip-hop, or any other style, you can learn about classes, clubs, competitions, and places to dance using the Internet. If you don't know where to look, try a search with the style of dance you're looking for and see what pops up.

After you're proficient, the Web can be your teacher by providing choreography and instruction, believe it or not! Here are some samples of online choreography sources.

Get Lively with Line Dancing

Tush Push. All Shook Up. Alley Cat. Walkin' Wazi. Country western line dancing is an energetic dance form that is popular all over the country. If you haven't seen it, the dancers are all in rows doing identical footwork, and at a certain moment, everyone knows to turn 90 or 180 degrees and start the dance again from another direction! It only looks like magic—the fact is that everyone learned the choreography. How many dances are there? More than 7,000, according to choreography site Kick It (`http://www.kickit.to`) where you can search by dance name, choreographer, or song. But don't worry, start by taking lessons, learn the most popular line dances in your area, and soon you'll find yourself on your feet all evening. Bonus for singles: One reason that line dancing is so popular is that you don't need a partner—you just get up and join the crowd.

Ballroom

`http://www.ballroomdancers.com`

Use this Web site to "explore the world of ballroom dancing, learn a new step, improve your technique, find a teacher or a partner, or ask a question about anything dance-related." You can even take a virtual lesson, such as how to move your hips Latin style (see Figure 9.2).

East Coast Swing

`http://www.dancetv.com/tutorial/swing/index.html`

Who needs a class when this site gives you a beginning series of swing lessons online, including little footprint illustrations to show you where your feet go on which beat?

West Coast Swing

`http://home.att.net/~wolfnyc/`

A New York City instructor teaches leader's patterns and variations, so you can really impress your follower.

Figure 9.2

BallroomDancers.com offers tips on technique, teachers, competitions, and other dance-related topics.

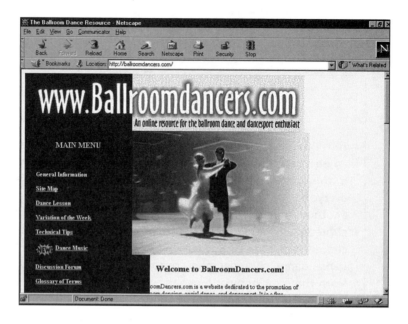

Fitness with the Family

We've already told you about the benefits of regular exercise and how staying in shape can help you keep up with your kids. But exercising *with* your family gives you the chance to spend quality time together and squeeze your workout into your busy schedule.

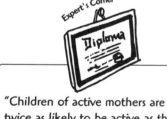

"Children of active mothers are twice as likely to be active as the children of inactive moms, and active dads are three-and-a-half times more likely to have active kids than sedentary dads are."

—Susan Kalish, executive director of the American Running Association, http://www.americanrunning.org

With only about half of Americans aged 12 to 21 regularly participating in vigorous physical activity, and studies revealing that childhood obesity is on the rise, it's up to parents to set a good example when it comes to fitness. Children learn by emulating their adult role models—if you're a channel surfer, that's the habit your child is going to pick up.

Instead, your children might even inspire you to get fit. Is your daughter interested in an activity you've always been curious about—say swimming or karate lessons? Why not join her and make it a family affair? When your child sees you fall down, get up, and try again, she learns that everyone has to make an effort—and that effort is an important part of life.

Family fitness activities also provide a way for parents to stay in touch with uncommunicative teenagers. Walking, inline skating, or biking, for example, all offer opportunities for nonconfrontational, casual conversation. During these activities, you can talk to your teens when the mood is light and without direct eye contact, making them feel more at ease and often more willing to open up. It really is true that "the family that plays together stays together!"

Encourage family fitness activities that are fun for everyone. First, talk to your children to find out what they would be interested in—don't try to choose an activity and "force" the family to join in. You can try traditional games such as baseball, basketball, or kickball, or make a day of it with cycling, swimming, hiking, camping, or canoeing. And don't forget the pleasures of a simple walk, a game of Frisbee, or raking leaves on a crisp autumn day—all these activities are sure to make you work up a sweat. For more ideas, check out the following Web sites.

99 Tips for Family Fitness Fun

    http://www.shapeup.org/publications/99.tips.for.family.fitness.fun/
    index.html

Shape Up America offers tips on family fitness at home, in the kitchen, at school, in the great outdoors, and in your own backyard.

365 Outdoor Activities

    http://family.go.com/Categories/Activities/Features/family_0401_01/
    dony/donyout_index/

From the "Acorn Toss" to the homemade "Water Slide," this site, excerpted from the book by Steve and Ruth Bennett, offers a multitude of ideas for fun and fitness outdoors.

Benny Goodsport

    http://www.bennygoodsport.com/

This is a great site for young children and parents to explore together. Take the Food Pyramid Challenge or read the Kickball Madness adventure story (see Figure 9.3).

Sports Parents

    http://www.sportsparents.com/

Info on equipment, coaching, training, and nutrition from Sports Illustrated for Kids.

Figure 9.3

Benny Goodsport shows kids how to get active and stay fit.

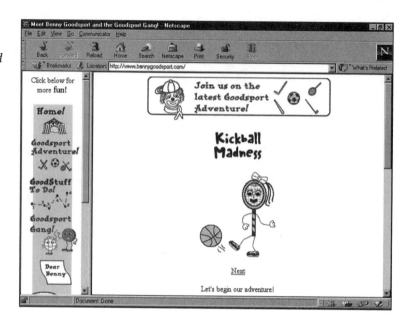

The Least You Need to Know

➤ You can have fun outdoors and get a great workout at the same time.

➤ Dancing is a top-notch way to combine exercise and social enjoyment.

➤ Planning family fitness activities is a wonderful way to spend quality time with your family and set a healthy example for your children.

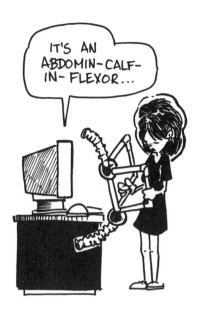

Chapter 10

Fitness Shopping on the Web: Equipment and Accessories

In This Chapter

➤ Determining what exercise equipment is right for your needs

➤ Using the Internet to research fitness equipment and accessories

➤ Shopping safely and avoiding scams online

One of the most useful and convenient applications of the Internet is at-home shopping. It's like a scene from "The Jetsons": Just sit down at your computer, tell it what you want, and it's delivered to your doorstep! But before you take advantage of this space-age technology, you've got to find the right type of exercise equipment and be sure you are purchasing it from a reputable source. This chapter shows you how. This chapter also shows you how to do your research on the Web, even if you decide to buy locally.

What Type of Equipment Do You Need?

There are hundreds of different fitness products you can use for your home workout—or to supplement your health-club membership on those days when you just can't make it to the gym. Finding these products is easy, because there are thousands of companies out there who want to sell them to you. But finding the right product from a reputable dealer on the Web can be more challenging than an advanced kick-boxing workout.

Maybe you've been suckered in by a celebrity-filled infomercial and bought a piece of equipment that now serves as a coat rack. Maybe you've purchased some fitness items on the advice of a friend, only to find out that these products don't motivate you or help you achieve your goals. If you can't or won't work out in a health club, how do you decide what exercise equipment you need in your home?

A recent Fitness Products Council study found that 50 million households nationwide own some type of fitness equipment, but nearly one-third of the equipment is gathering dust in a corner. Too many people buy exercise equipment impulsively and end up with something that accomplishes nothing but embarrassing them as they walk by it several times a day.

Before making a major equipment purchase, figure out your fitness goals and pin down what fitness activities you really enjoy. If you want to lose weight, a treadmill is a better choice than a home gym. If you don't like bike riding, no stationary cycle is going to motivate you to work out at home. If you think stair-stepping is a bore at the club, it won't ring your chimes any better at home.

If you're buying a major piece of equipment—a cardio machine or a home gym—please don't purchase it without trying it, even if what you've found on the Web sounds swell. You wouldn't buy a car without test driving it, or marry a man without dating him. A good piece of exercise equipment is a major financial investment and time commitment, so you need to be sure that model is one you'll be happy to use, day after day after day.

So, do your research on the Web, but it's usually a good idea to buy big-ticket items from a local exercise-equipment specialty store. You can try and compare different models, and you can get local servicing if you need it.

Go to the store in workout clothes, get on the machine, and work out while you ask the salesperson a billion questions. If you don't enjoy ten minutes on this machine in the store, how do you expect to look forward to your workout daily?

For tips on purchasing exercise equipment, take a look at the following sites:

Avoiding the Muscle Hustle: Tips for Buying Exercise Equipment

```
http://www.ftc.gov/bcp/conline/edcams/exercise/index.html
```

Making a fitness equipment purchase is a major commitment. Don't get taken in by outrageous advertising claims. This site helps you become a better informed consumer (see Figure 10.1).

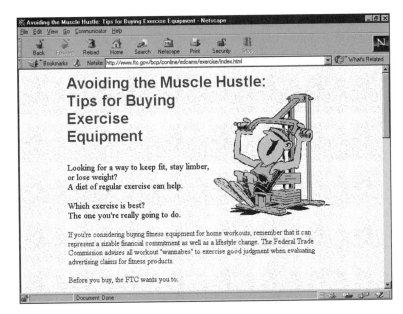

10 Tips for Purchasing Fitness Equipment

`http://www.fitathome.com/howtobuy.htm`

Know yourself, analyze your space, and buy from a reputable dealer. These are a few of the tips offered by the Fitness Products Council and Web store Fit @ Home.

Buying Home Cardio Equipment: Where to Shop and What to Ask

`http://www.fitnesslink.com/homegym/buyhome.htm`

Joan offers solid advice on what to look for when buying home cardio exercise equipment from a retail store, and why to choose a specialty store.

Choosing and Using Exercise Equipment

`http://www.quackwatch.com/03HealthPromotion/eqpt.html`

This article, reprinted by Quackwatch from *The Physician and Sportsmedicine*, presents questions to ask yourself to help you select the right variety of exercise equipment, and then some facts on choosing a good treadmill, stationary bike, rower, cross-country skier, stair-stepper, or exercise rider.

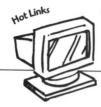

Hot Links

How to Shop for a Treadmill

http://www.montana.com/Stafford/treadmill.html

If you really get serious about buying a treadmill, here's the scoop on horsepower, belts, motor torque, warranties, and everything you need to know to make an intelligent choice. Print this out and take it to the store with you.

Finding Fitness Products Online

There are enough companies selling fitness products online to keep you surfing for weeks. If you know the brand, you can do a search for that company's Web site. If you're not sure what you want, start with these super sites that will help you find whatever product you seek.

Start Here: Equipment for Sale

If you do decide to buy online, the following sites are examples of reputable exercise-equipment sites that offer information as well as products.

Fit @ Home

http://www.fitathome.com

Choose from a wide selection of home gyms, cardio equipment, resistance tubes, exercise balls, videos, free weights, and accessories such as weightlifting gloves and belts. The "Fitness Club" section of this site offers a fitness FAQ, a discussion board, a personal trainer locator, fitness articles and tips, and links to fitness information sites.

Fogdog Sports

http://www.fogdog.com

Shop by sport or by brand name to find loads of fitness products and sporting goods. Many sport sections have their own "experts" offering product purchasing guidelines and sport-related advice.

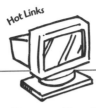

Fitness Registry

```
http://www.fitnessregistry.com
```

This is a directory of specialty fitness equipment stores. Use the Fitness Registry's searchable Web site to find a specialty fitness store near you. Or use Retail Links to find the Web sites of exercise-equipment dealers on the Internet.

The Internet's Fitness Resource: Equipment and Clothing Links

```
http://www.netsweat.com/equipap.htm
```

This links site puts you in touch with many kinds of fitness equipment sellers on the Web—from the manufacturer to the retailer.

Yahoo!'s Equipment Manufacturer's Links

```
http://dir.yahoo.com/Business_and_Economy/Companies/Health/Fitness/
Exercise_Equipment/Manufacturers/
```

Yahoo! links you to many of the major fitness equipment manufacturers, from Aqua Trend to Z-Lift.

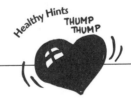

Dyna-Band Workout

Do you wish you had some exercise equipment that was versatile, effective, traveled easily, and weighed almost nothing? Dyna-Bands are stretchy latex strips that work the muscles like weights, but take practically no storage space and can travel tucked into a pocket. You can keep them by the computer for stretch-and-strengthen breaks, take them on trips, or store them in a desk drawer at work. Buy Dyna-Bands from Joan's business, Unconventional Moves, by phoning toll-free 1-888-BFITTER or emailing jprice@sonic.net. Free illustrated instructions are included.

Exercise Videos

Would you enjoy working out with celebrities or world-class instructors? Don't limit yourself to the few exercise videotapes you find at your local stores—choose from hundreds as you browse or buy at these specialty sites.

Video Fitness

http://www.videofitness.com

This incredibly useful site is a gold mine of information. It includes reviews of just about every exercise video in existence, written by people just like you. Check out fun features, such as "Desert Island Videos" (if you were stranded on a desert island, what five exercise videos would you have to have?), the "Hall of Fame" (videos that have received over ten favorable reviews), tips for beginners, and the active bulletin board.

Collage Video

http://www.collagevideo.com

Collage Video offers a free catalog that reviews and sells more than 400 exercise videos, and they've been doing it for 12 years. All the reviews are written by people who have actually done the workouts. If you're not sure what you want, you can phone and they'll help you figure out what you'd enjoy based on your fitness level, exercise experience, and preferences.

Active Videos

http://www.activevideos.com/

Active Videos offers a diverse range of dance (swing, funk, square, ballroom, jazz, and more) and sports (including inline skating, cheerleading, and football) exercise videos, in addition to the traditional "aerobics" videos (see Figure 10.2).

Amazon.com

http://www.amazon.com

Yes, the major online bookseller also has hundreds of workout videos, most with descriptive reviews to help you decide what to buy. Click **video**, then **special interests**, and then **fitness**. You can view the top 75 bestsellers, or do a search for the title, instructor, or category you want.

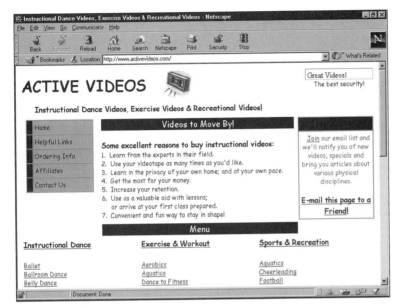

Figure 10.2

The Active Videos Web site is packed with "videos to move by."

Monitors and Calipers

A heart monitor tells you how intensely you're exercising. Calipers help you judge the amount of body fat you're carrying. You can buy both on the Web.

Polar Heart Rate Monitors

```
http://www.polar.fi
```

Information and support for Polar's heart rate monitors can be found on this site. Type some info about yourself to use their "personal trainer" feature, offering fitness tips and a workout guide.

Tanita

```
http://www.tanita.com/02_main_menu.html
```

Tanita offers high-tech scales and body fat monitors. Their site includes complete details on their products as well as "tips and tools for weight and body fat management."

Body Caliper

```
http://www.bodycaliper.com
```

The Body Caliper offers a body fat testing device to help you determine whether your workout is resulting in fat loss and muscle gain.

Shopping Online—Is It Safe?

After you've determined the product you want and located the company you want to buy from, you usually have two choices: Buy online or buy through traditional channels (over the phone or by sending in a check). You might be concerned about giving your credit card number out online, but technology now exists that makes online shopping as safe as shopping by phone. And if you ever have a problem, you can simply dispute the charge by writing your credit card company.

Look for a site that offers "secure" purchasing. This means that when you enter your credit card number into an order form, it is scrambled, or "encrypted," and then decoded when it is received by the company. There is a slim chance that some high-techie or "hacker" could get your credit-card number while it is being transmitted from your computer to the Web-store's computer. But according to Yahoo! (http://www.yahoo.com), the giant Web directory, and host of a slew of online store-fronts, "If you are not the kind of person who worries about being hit by lightning as you're crossing the street, you probably don't have to worry that your credit card number will be intercepted on the way to a secure Web site."

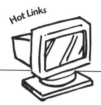

Hot Links

The Public Eye

http://www.thepubliceye.com

The Public Eye "certifies" Web merchants and keeps a record of reports that are filed by their customers. The system monitors online stores for reliability, privacy, and customer satisfaction, and the reports are immediately available to other consumers.

Use the PILOT method when searching for online shopping sites. A quality online store not only sells you a product, but also offers useful information, links, and timely updates of pricing and inventory. Check out the company's warranty and return policies—they should be readily available on the Web site. The company's physical address and phone number should be displayed on the site. If you can't identify where they are, move on to the next store.

Count to Ten (or 100) Before Purchasing the Latest "Gadget"

If you're tempted to buy a gadget or gizmo, realize it's probably a gimmick. These silly excuses for equipment use fantastic claims to lure you in—trim your thighs with this one little piece of plastic, blast your abdominals with no effort whatsoever, firm that saggy butt in two minutes a week…it just goes on and on.

Investigate first: What is the product really, how does it work, what research studies (not testimonials!) confirm that it works. Read impartial reviews from outside sources. (For more, read Joan's articles on money-wasters on FitnessLink. Start at `http://www.joanprice.com` and scroll to the list of articles. Then select **Save Your Bucks: Exercise Money-Wasters**, **Quack Alert**, and **Abdominal Devices**.)

The Least You Need to Know

➤ You should determine your fitness goals and home workout needs before purchasing exercise equipment.

➤ The Internet is a tremendous resource when shopping for fitness equipment and accessories—but you must be aware of the scams that abound online.

➤ You might want to research online and buy locally if you're making a large equipment purchase.

➤ Shopping online is generally safe when buying from a reputable dealer.

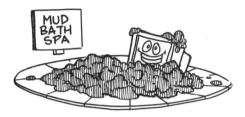

Chapter 11

Hit the Road: Health and Fitness Resorts, Spas, and Vacations

In This Chapter

➤ Learning how to take your fitness habit on the road

➤ Taking active vacations to promote your fitness habit

➤ Finding a spa or resort vacation using the Internet

➤ Finding a hotel with a gym

Do you return home from a vacation or business trip more tired than when you left? Do you find yourself regretting the opulent meals and sluggish habits you indulged in? Do you dread stepping on the scales the Monday morning after your return? Do you beat yourself up for abandoning your exercise habit while you were away?

It doesn't have to happen! Instead of lying at the pool, guzzling beer, and snacking on chips, you can treat your body and your mind to an exhilarating fitness adventure. You *can* take your fitness habit on the road with you, whether you're traveling for business or pleasure, and the World Wide Web can help you do it. This chapter shows you how.

Treat Yourself to a Healthy Vacation!

The word "vacation" means different things to different people. Whether you enjoy a relaxing cruise, a week at the beach, or a vigorous camping and hiking trip, you can get fitness benefits on your vacation.

Taking Your Fitness Habit with You

Staying fit on a vacation or business trip is easy if you plan for it. If you exercise first thing in the morning when you're at home, plan to keep that schedule. If you're used to exercising on your way home from work, plan your workout at that same time of day—your body is expecting it. Pack athletic shoes, a tank top, and shorts that you can rinse out in the sink and dry quickly, and sweats if the weather might be cool.

In the olden days (before all these services went online), you had to wait until you got to your destination to find out about the running or cycling routes or where to rent skates or bikes. Now you can do this all online.

Do a search on your destination city and "fitness" or the specific activity you are interested in, "biking," for example. After wading through the links with some patience, you'll find information on your chosen activity, along with an assortment of health clubs, personal trainers, martial arts classes, running clubs, hiking trails, and so on. Another way to go is to choose the online Yellow Pages and search by city and category (fitness, skating, health clubs, tai chi, whatever interests you).

Ask the locals. If you're looking for a running trail or cycling route, a good bet is to use the online Yellow Pages to find a store that specializes in that sport (a running-shoe store or bicycle shop), and phone or email to ask for information. Runners love to help other runners enjoy their cities, and the friendly cyclist in the bike shop might invite you to join the local cycling club for a ride.

Dyna-Bands to Go

Your strength-training program doesn't have to bite the dust when you're traveling. Dyna-Bands are stretchy, three-foot-long, latex bands made specifically for strengthening and stretching. They come in four different resistance levels and work your muscles as though you're lifting weights. Dyna-Bands weigh only ounces and tuck into a pocket for traveling. Dyna-Bands are available from Joan's business, Unconventional Moves. To order, call toll-free 888-BFITTER (888-234-8837) or email jprice@sonic.net. A free, illustrated routine is included with each order.

Become an Active Vacationer

If your yearly vacation always involves lying on a beach reading a book, why not add some spice to your life with an active or adventure vacation? Ski the Rockies. Cycle across your state. Hike a portion of the Appalachian Trail. Scuba dive in the Caribbean. Kayak the Colorado River. Treat your mind and body to a fitness spa retreat. You don't need to be an athlete to enjoy adventure travel—you just need to thrive on being active and enjoy being outdoors. Search for "adventure travel" with your favorite search tool, or check out these online sites to get fired up for a new experience.

Country Walkers

http://countrywalkers.com/countrywalkers/welcome.htm

"Explore the world... one step at a time." Guided tours offer walkers the opportunity to enjoy scenic landscapes and explore small towns (see Figure 11.1).

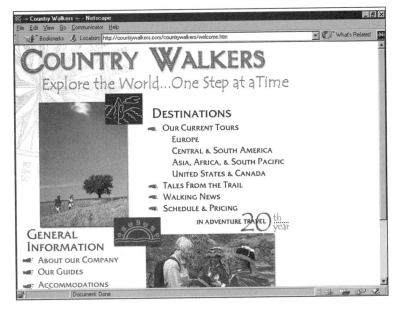

Figure 11.1

Country Walkers takes you down "the road less traveled."

America by Bicycle

http://www.abbike.com

You can see the country from the seat of your bicycle.

Ski Travel Online

http://www.skito.com

Ski Travel Online provides destination details and online booking for tons of ski resorts. In the summer months, this site becomes "Mountain Travel Online."

O.A.R.S.: The Outdoor Adventure River Specialists

http://www.oars.com

O.A.R.S. offers river vacations that are "a medley of fun and excitement, relaxation, and serenity." Search their Trip Finder, get details on more than 50 itineraries, and visit their Online River Store to get your gear.

Worldwide Outdoor Adventures

http://www.wwoutdooradventures.com/

"Your one-stop outdoor recreation and adventure specialist." Here you'll find details on rafting, hunting, fishing, golfing—even safari vacations! Email or call to book all your travel arrangements through them.

Outward Bound

http://www.outwardbound.com

The challenge of surviving in the wilderness, the support and camaraderie of a team. Learn wilderness skills and put them to use. "You might lead an ascent, captain a boat, or navigate through difficult terrain."

Women's Quest Fitness Camps

http://www.womensquest.com

"Come out and play." These camps in Colorado and Vermont aim to strengthen body, mind, and spirit and empower women of all athletic abilities. Their retreats "combine physical, mindful, and spirit-filled activities with challenging adventures that encourage personal awareness and self-expression." Activities are noncompetitive and appropriate for a range of abilities—"from beginning walkers to seasoned triathletes."

Club Med

http://www.clubmed.com/

If you want a good dose of fun, entertainment, and lively social interaction along with physical activity, you might enjoy a Club Med vacation. Golf, scuba diving, tennis, horseback riding—choose a destination that matches your favored sport.

Crunch Your Abs

Abdominal crunches—also called curl-ups—can be done anywhere, including hotel rooms. Lie on your back, knees bent, feet flat on the floor. Cross your arms over your chest or place your hands behind your neck, elbows out to the side. Do not pull on your head. Take a deep breath. As you exhale, pull your abdominal muscles in and let that muscle contraction lift your chest, then shoulders, and then—if you're strong enough—shoulder blades. Hold at the top for two seconds before slowly releasing down. Keep your head and neck relaxed through the whole sequence. Do as many as you can in good form. Work up to five minutes of crunches if you're strong enough, but even one or two minutes will make a difference if you do these regularly.

Finding a Resort or Spa on the Web

For a vacation—or just a weekend getaway—filled with low-fat gourmet cuisine, challenging fitness classes, adventurous outdoor activities, massages, steam showers, facials, and other rejuvenating personal services, look into visiting a spa or resort.

Think of the Internet as your personal travel agent, available 24 hours a day at the click of a mouse. Your computer can take the stress out of finding the perfect spa or resort vacation. Instead of spending days researching destinations, requesting brochures, and waiting for them to arrive by mail, and then phoning various resorts to get your questions answered, all this information is available at your fingertips. The following sites are a few good places to start.

The Spa Source

```
http://www.spafinders.com
```

Search the world of spas at this Web site. The Spa-Finder allows you to search for fitness resorts by category, interest, or location. You'll also find articles from the Spa-Finder Newsletter and a few spa recipes so you can prepare healthy resort-style food in your own kitchen.

Spa Magazine

```
http://www.spamagazine.com
```

You can search by state or category for resorts and day spas worldwide. This site includes articles from Spa Magazine, many dealing with health and fitness (see Figure 11.2).

Figure 11.2

Spa Magazine's Web site helps you search for spas worldwide.

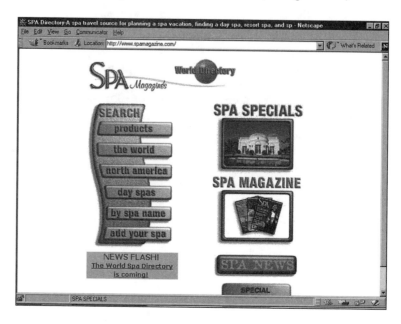

Traveling for Business or Pleasure: Finding a Hotel with a Gym

Nowadays, many hotels have gyms—or at least they have little locked rooms they call gyms. The equipment varies from "Wow, I wish I had this at home!" to "I'm supposed to work out on *that*?" Usually, you'll find at least free weights or a multistation weight machine, a treadmill or stair machine, and maybe an exercise bike. Even if the facility is not state-of-the-art, you can get a workout, and you'll have much more physical and mental energy if you do.

Some hotels have reciprocal arrangements with nearby health clubs, and although it means taking a short walk (you wanted to exercise, didn't you?), the facility is usually far superior to an onsite hotel gym. Plus you can take exercise classes, if that's your pleasure.

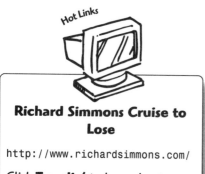

Richard Simmons Cruise to Lose

http://www.richardsimmons.com/

Click **Travelin'** to learn about Richard's seven-day cruises. You'll "sweat with the oldies," listen to Richard's motivating talks, eat healthy, and make new friends.

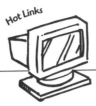

Hot Links

Travel Tips: Taking Your Fitness Habit on the Road

`http://www.joanprice.com`

Scroll through the list of Joan's articles until you find **Travel Tips**, and read about how to plan for an active vacation or business trip, including exercise suggestions. For even more, get Joan's book, *Joan Price Says, Yes, You CAN Get in Shape!*, and read the "Travel Fitness" chapter, with exercises you can do in the hotel, outdoors, and even in the car!

If you know where you want to stay, or you are making your travel arrangements online, most hotels have Web sites that list their amenities—just browse the hotel's site to see what they offer in terms of exercise facilities.

If you've ever arrived at a hotel that advertised a gym and found a rickety bike and an old multistation gym with half the weight pins missing, check out Fit for Business at `http://www.fitforbusiness.com` before making your reservations. This site evaluates hotel fitness centers. If you want to find a hotel gym with free weights or racquetball, or you want to know how many cardio machines a fitness center offers, you can look it up here. The listing is far from comprehensive, but you might get lucky and learn about a hotel with an exceptional gym in your city of choice. You don't have to be a business traveler to take advantage of these listings.

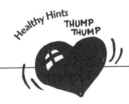

Healthy Hints

THUMP
THUMP

Safe Luggage Lifting

Nothing turns your vacation into a nightmare faster than hurting your back when lifting a suitcase, and this happens surprisingly often. Avoid a bum back by lifting properly: Keep your back straight and knees bent. Avoid twisting while lifting or carrying. Don't lift a suitcase that's too heavy—ask for help. A small investment that pays off big-time is a rolling luggage cart or a suitcase with wheels.

The Least You Need to Know

➤ Active and adventurous vacations can leave you feeling healthy and exhilarated.

➤ The Internet can be a valuable tool in researching your travel plans and providing new vacation ideas.

➤ You don't have to abandon your fitness habit when you travel.

Part 3

How to Find Nutrition, Diet, and Weight-Loss Information Online

The worlds of weight loss, diet, and nutrition are riddled with hoaxes, gimmicks, weirdness, and general confusion over what "works" and what doesn't. Losing weight and eating right are really no mystery—most credible experts agree on the basics— and the Internet is a valuable source for education and support.

If you want to understand nutrition, we've got the resources that make this subject make sense. If you're trying to lose weight, we steer you to sites that can help you do it the right way. You'll learn to recognize and avoid fad diets and the scams that prey on weight-loss hopefuls. We also encourage you to accept and enjoy your body exactly as it is. You'll learn how to use the Internet to make cooking a breeze. And whatever your goals—whether it's affirming positive body image, losing 20 pounds, or exchanging recipes—we'll hook you up with friends online who share them.

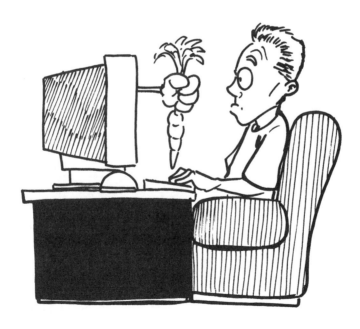

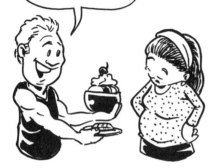

YOU CAN EAT ICE CREAM BUT YOU HAVE TO FOLLOW IT UP WITH 3 OUNCES OF SALMON.

Chapter 12

Nutrition 101: Sorting It Out

In This Chapter

➤ Understanding calories, carbohydrates, proteins, and fats

➤ Figuring out how to eat a healthy diet

➤ Creating your own diet plan with online help

How do you decipher what foods and food plans are good for you? It's about time you gave us an easy question. Among credible experts and organizations, there's little discord. This chapter tells you what the experts say about eating for health, and the Web sites you can use to educate and guide yourself.

You Are What You Eat

This isn't just another cliché—it's absolutely true. Eat a lot of fat and your body becomes fat. Stick mainly to fresh, wholesome fruits and vegetables and your body rewards you with healthful energy and a strong immune system.

Calories

It's a common question: "How many calories do I need?" Here's our uncommon answer: "It depends." It depends on your goal (whether it be weight loss, maintenance, or muscle gain), age, sex, current weight, personal metabolic rate, and your activity level.

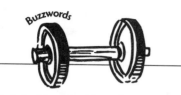

Metabolic rate: The calories you burn at rest, meaning the calories required to keep your organs working if you don't move a muscle all day. (We don't recommend that, however.)

In general, adult women need between 1,600 and 2,000 calories a day; adult men require 1,800 to 2,200 calories. But we don't really like generalities. To calculate your caloric needs, try this formula:

(Desired Body Weight) × (Activity Level Factor) = Total Daily Calorie Needs

Activity level factors:

12 = light activity

15 = moderate activity

18 = heavy activity

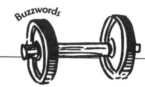

Calories: Technically, one calorie is the amount of heat necessary to raise the temperature of a liter of water one degree centigrade. Simply put, calories measure the energy produced by food in the body.

There are ways to calculate caloric need, and some are more comprehensive than others. We suggest you try the following online calorie calculators and take an average of your results, or stay within the range of your results.

Nutritional Profile from CyberDiet

```
http://www.CyberDiet.com/profile/profile.html
```

Why do the math when CyberDiet tells you how many calories you need based on your age, weight, gender, and activity level? Even better, decide what percentage of fat you're aiming for in your diet, and your nutritional profile tells you how many calories to eat; how many grams of protein, carbohydrates, and fat you need; and your vitamin, minerals, and fiber needs.

Mylifepath.com

```
http://www.mylifepath.com/topic/calneed
```

Brought to you by Blue Shield of California, this site's calorie calculator determines your needs and then follows it up with targeted recommendations to help you lose, gain, or maintain your weight (see Figure 12.1).

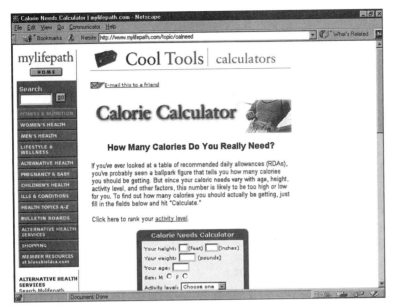

Figure 12.1

Determine your caloric needs at mylifepath.com.

Carbohydrates

Carbohydrates fuel the body. During digestion, carbohydrates breaks down into glucose, the body's most efficient and readily available energy source.

The most nutritious carbohydrates are the complex carbohydrates: starchy vegetables and grains such as rice, beans, potatoes, sweet potatoes, oats, green vegetables, and fruit. These are good sources of fiber, which is important for health and for prevention of disease. There are also simple carbohydrates, such as sweets and baked goods made from refined sugars, that provide little more than empty calories.

Carbohydrate foods contain four calories per gram. The latest research recommends the average adult get 55 to 70 percent of their daily calories from high-quality carbohydrates.

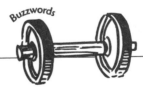

Buzzwords

Fiber: Fiber is a type of carbohydrate that is indigestible. It passes through your digestive system, helping to move other contents along. A high-fiber diet promotes a feeling of fullness, prevents various intestinal problems, and might reduce your risk of heart disease. See "How to Increase the Amount of Fiber in Your Diet" at `http://www.aafp.org/patientinfo/fiber.html`.

125

Proteins

Proteins are essential for the growth and repair of all body tissues. Unlike carbohydrates and fats, proteins are not an efficient source of energy, and are used for energy only in extreme cases when no carbohydrate or fat is available.

The average American diet provides plenty of protein, as it is abundant in meat and dairy products. Beans are also an excellent source of protein—especially for the vegetarian.

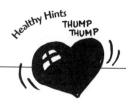

Healthy Hints THUMP THUMP

Bean Bonanza

Doctors and nutritionists alike recognize the high nutritional value of beans. The USDA's Food Guide Booklet recommends one-half cup of beans as a protein substitute for one ounce of meat. Beans are a good source of dietary fiber and B vitamins and are fat-free and low in calories—making them a tasty and healthful addition to any meal. They're inexpensive and versatile and can be used in many ways to complement a meal.

Protein foods contain four calories per gram. The average adult needs 15 to 25 percent of their daily calories from protein.

Fats

Fats are the black sheep of the food pyramid family. Usually referred to in terms of saturated and unsaturated, all types of fat contribute to the development of a variety of diseases, most notably heart disease.

Fats are the most concentrated source of food energy at nine calories per gram. Although the American Heart Association recommends that no more than 30 percent of your calories come from fat, other medical experts recommend you go lower than that. Some experts, such as Dean Ornish, M.D. (http://www.ornish.com), and John McDougall, M.D. (http://drmcdougall.com/), say that 10 percent is ideal for heart health and weight management. They would like us to cut out all dietary fat except what is naturally in plant-based foods (no added oil, no animal products). Other experts say that we're too obsessed about fat and just need to concern ourselves with balance and nutritious food choices.

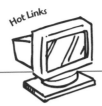

Hot Links

Fatfree: The Low-Fat Vegetarian Recipe Archive,
http://www.fatfree.com

This site contains a searchable database of more than 2,500 vegetarian recipes in more than 50 categories, including soups, casseroles, desserts, regional foods, and many more. You don't have to be a full-time vegetarian to enjoy these recipes. The site includes a link to the USDA nutrient database—another excellent site—which provides nutrient listings for tons of foods. Search for your food to get the breakdown of fat, protein, carbohydrate, vitamin, mineral, cholesterol, sodium, fiber, and more nutritional information.

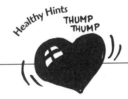

Healthy Hints   THUMP THUMP

Understanding Fats

➤ **Saturated Fat**   Solid at room temperature. The most saturated fats are butter, palm kernel oil, and coconut oil. Saturated fat is considered the greatest health risk because it raises blood cholesterol and clogs arteries.

➤ **Polyunsaturated Fat**   Liquid at room temperature. Polyunsaturated fats include corn and soybean oils, fish oils, sesame oil, and sunflower oil. Recent research has shown that polyunsaturated fats lower the "good" HDL cholesterol and might increase risk for certain types of cancer.

➤ **Monounsaturated Fat**   Also liquid at room temperature, monounsaturated fats, such as olive oil and canola oil, lower the "bad" LDL cholesterol and maintain the "good" HDL cholesterol levels. This is the fat to choose—if you have to choose any!

➤ **Hydrogenated Fats**   Also known as trans fatty acids, these fats are unnaturally manufactured by adding hydrogen to liquid oils to make them semisolid. Essentially, this process takes an unsaturated fat and turns it into a saturated fat.

One thing is certain: Americans are getting fatter. Even though we are eating more "low-fat" and "fat-free" foods, we are still eating more fat, and more calories, than we should.

Each body is different, and you might need to experiment with different healthy (not fad!) amounts of fat to find what makes you feel healthy and vigorous. Joan thrives on a very low-fat vegan diet, while Shannon feels best with a slightly higher fat and protein level.

Other healthy, fit people might have distinctly different eating styles. But please don't trust anyone who recommends that you can eat all the fat you want—we know that's harmful to your health.

Vitamins and Minerals

What vitamins and minerals do we need? How much? Which foods contain them? Do we have to take supplements? The Web has unlimited vitamin information. It also has unlimited pseudoinformation, too—so, please remember the PILOT Method! Here are some good sites that will answer all your questions.

Vitamins Network

http://www.vitamins.net

Click **Guide to Vitamins**, which presents the benefits, RDA, best food sources, synergistic nutrients, deficiency symptoms, and negative interactions of each vitamin and mineral.

Vitamins and Minerals from The Food and Nutrition Information Center (FNIC)

http://www.nal.usda.gov/fnic/etext/000068.html#v&m

This page has links to other sites' reputable articles on an array of vitamins and minerals. The FNIC is part of the United States Department of Agriculture (USDA).

Vitamin and Nutritional Supplements: Sorting Out Fact from Fiction amid a Storm of Controversy

http://www.mayohealth.org/mayo/9707/htm/me_jun97.htm

The nutritional supplement industry is a $6 billion-a-year business. This article from the Mayo Clinic's Health Oasis helps you cut through the hype to understand just what you need and why.

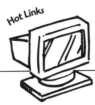

Hot Links

American Dietetic Association (ADA)

`http://www.eatright.org/`

The 70,000 members of the ADA are food and nutrition professionals—75 percent are registered dietitians (RDs). Click **Nutrition Resources** link to find a collection of simple tips, features, and book excerpts to help you improve your eating habits. You can locate a registered dietitian in your area by clicking the **Find a Dietitian** link from the home page.

What Exactly Is a "Healthy Diet"?

The major health/dietary organizations have joined hands on this one to issue the Unified Dietary Guidelines, which you can read about on FitnessLink at `http://www.fitnesslink.com/nutrition/udg.htm`.

The new guidelines are a straightforward master plan of exactly what foods you're supposed to eat to be your healthiest. Four primary health organizations—the American Cancer Society, the American Dietetic Association, the American Academy of Pediatrics, and the National Institutes of Health—have endorsed an eating plan that helps prevent some of the killer diseases: heart disease, stroke, cancer, and diabetes. By presenting a unified plan, nutrition experts hope to clear up the misunderstandings that abound about diet. They also hope to drive home the message that yes, diet affects health, and here's how to take advantage of what we know.

So, what's the message? We need to cut down on fat (especially saturated fat), sugar, salt, and calories. We need to eat more fruits, vegetables and low-fat products. (Big surprise?) The new guidelines include:

➤ Eat a variety of foods.

➤ Eat five or more servings of fruits and vegetables each day.

➤ Choose most of what you eat from plant sources.

➤ Eat six or more servings of bread, pasta, and cereal grains each day.

➤ Reduce the amount of high-fat foods, especially those from animal sources.

➤ Minimize sweets.

The bottom line: You can't go wrong eating a healthy diet composed of naturally low-fat, high-fiber foods, such as fruits, vegetables, and grains.

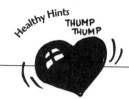

Wisdom of the Pyramid

A useful plan for making healthy food choices is the Food Guide Pyramid, endorsed by the American Dietetic Association, which puts no foods off limits, but advises you to eat more of some food types, less of others. Here are the recommendations:

➤ **Bread, cereal, rice, pasta**   6–11 servings

➤ **Vegetables**   3–5 servings

➤ **Fruit**   2–4 servings

➤ **Meat, poultry, fish, dry beans, eggs, nuts**   2–3 servings

➤ **Milk, yogurt, cheese**   2–3 servings

➤ **Fats, oils, sweets**   Use sparingly.

You can find the Food Guide Pyramid online at `http://www.nal.usda.gov:8001/py/pmap.htm` (see Figure 12.2). The American Dietetic Association explains the Pyramid—what to eat, how much (including how to figure out what a "serving" is), and how to eat a variety of foods to get the nutrients and calories you need to maintain a healthy weight. You can click each section of the pyramid for more information. This handy guide shows you the most sensible way to eat healthy.

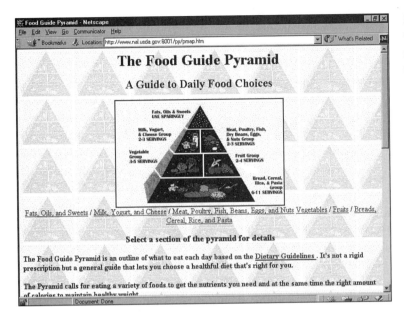

Figure 12.2

The Food Guide Pyramid makes healthy eating easy.

Online Advice Abounds

Nutrition news is notoriously confusing. You make a serious effort to include a specific food in your diet because a study says it's the new "wonder food," only to hear a few months later that your wonder food is now considered poison. Nutrition information online is no different, and is probably even more suspect, because virtually anyone can get on the Internet and call themselves "experts."

Be critical of sites that cite new findings uncovered by recent "studies." Just because one study suggests the benefits of a certain food or type of diet, it doesn't mean you should take this as gospel. Many of these "studies" are conducted with a very small number of people. Many are paid for by a corporation with a decided interest in the outcome. Look for the specifics before subscribing to a new diet philosophy.

When surfing through online nutrition advice, keep the basics we outlined in this chapter in mind. If you come across something radically different, scrutinize the information carefully. Who are the "experts" offering this nutrition advice? Do they have an agenda? A product to sell?

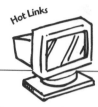

Nutrition News Focus

http://www.nutritionnewsfocus.com/

NNF provides a daily email newsletter that helps you "make sense of all the confusing nutrition news you're bombarded with every day." The Web site displays archives of the newsletter and is chock-full of concise explanations of the latest nutrition news. This news is brought to you by Dr. David Klurfeld, Professor and Chairman of the Department of Nutrition and Food Science at Wayne State University in Detroit and Editor in Chief of the *Journal of the American College of Nutrition*. The newsletter is free and it doesn't have anything to sell—those involved just want to help you better understand nutrition news.

Start Here

For a wealth of nutrition information, you can't go wrong with these special sites.

Tufts Nutrition Navigator

http://navigator.tufts.edu

Tufts provides links to the cream-of-the-crop nutrition Web sites (see Figure 12.3). An excellent place to start your search for nutrition information online, their professional advisory board reviews each site and rates them on the basis of accuracy, depth of information, how up-to-date the information is, and the overall "user experience" (similar to our PILOT method).

Mayo Clinic Health Oasis Nutrition Center

http://www2.mayohealth.org/mayo/common/htm/dietpage.htm

This is a great playground if you're interested in health and nutrition, or just like to read about food. A registered dietitian answers questions, such as the nutrition and calories in sushi and game meats (not in the same meal, please). A "Virtual Cookbook" gives you the both the traditional recipe and a healthier modification for hundreds of both familiar and esoteric menu items, including the nutritional breakdown of the "before" and "after." Reference articles cover subjects as varied as cooking for one and the connection between food and disease prevention. This is one of our top choices for solid and interesting nutrition information. It passes our PILOT test with flying colors!

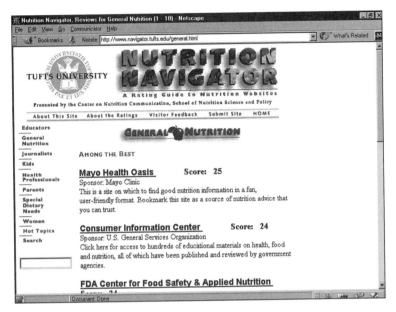

Figure 12.3

Tufts Nutrition Navigator rates nutrition Web sites based on accuracy, depth, currency, and usability.

Center for Science in the Public Interest

http://www.cspinet.org

CSPI, a nutrition advocacy organization, focuses on improving the safety and nutritional quality of our food supply. When you're ready to go beyond nutrition basics, you can find a wealth of information about food safety, additives, junk foods (for example, soft drinks are called "liquid candy"), as well as revelations about foods, food substitutes, and restaurant options that are hazardous to your health. Nutrition quizzes, excerpts from the Nutrition Action Health Letter, and links to other nutrition Web sites abound.

Veggies Unite!

http://www.vegweb.com

If you're a vegetarian or vegan, this site must be bookmarked on your browser! A storehouse of quality information, Veggies Unite! offers more than 3,000 vegan recipes, a vitamin and mineral guide, links to veggie-related articles on the Web, a grocery list maker, a weekly meal planner, and much more.

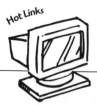

Hot Links

Blonz Guide to Nutrition, Food & Health Resources

`http://www.blonz.com/`

Compiled by Ed Blonz, Ph.D., a nutrition consultant and author, the Blonz Guide is a vast collection of links to nutrition, food, food science, fitness, and medical and health sites. Blonz also provides links to government agencies, newspapers, and health and medical publications, as well as links to the nutrition departments of several university Web sites.

The Least You Need to Know

➤ The ideal diet is balanced, varied, and nutritious.

➤ Use the Food Guide Pyramid to plan healthy meals.

➤ Eat more high-fiber carbohydrates and less sugar, fat, and highly processed foods.

➤ Several Web sites can help you make informed food choices that contribute to a healthier you.

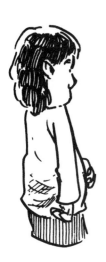
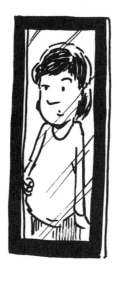

Chapter 13

It's No Mystery: Losing Weight Safely and Effectively

In This Chapter

➤ Understanding how weight loss happens—and doesn't happen

➤ Making food choices for optimal nutrition and lasting weight loss

➤ Figuring out your realistic weight goal

➤ Finding reliable online sources of weight-loss information

To use the Web successfully for your weight-loss program, you must seek out reliable information and push away the thousands of gimmicky sites that insist they've discovered the permanent, secret, breakthrough, new, or ancient weight-loss solution.

Realize this: These folks have a product or a plan to sell, and you need to screen their products as carefully as you would an elixir hawked by a door-to-door salesman or at a booth at the fair. This chapter helps you grab onto the facts and kick away the fiction of weight loss, saving you money, frustration, and grief.

The Business of Weight Loss

Joan calls January "National Shape-Up Month," because as a personal trainer specializing in helping non- and lapsed exercisers, she gets more calls from new clients and the media in January than any other three months combined. People look at themselves in the mirror after a holiday season of indulging and yowl, "What have I done?" Millions resolve to lose weight. A few months later, most give up and regain the weight they've lost—if any. Even so, weight loss remains a goal and weight-loss failure remains an embarrassment.

At any time of the year, 15 to 35 percent of Americans are trying to drop pounds of flesh, spending $30 billion to $50 billion yearly. About 80 percent of Americans have tried an average of four weight-loss methods apiece over the past year.

If most of these methods worked, we wouldn't have to keep trying the same or different ones over and over again! The truth is that most don't work. You won't find any quick fixes in this chapter, because quick fixes are fakes. Learn that lesson, and you're halfway to success. The other half comes from understanding what does work.

Calories In, Calories Out

What do the U.S. Department of Agriculture, the American Heart Association, the American Dietetic Association, and the American Medical Association all have in common? They agree that the most realistic and successful approach to weight loss is to eat a balanced diet of a variety of foods in moderate amounts, and follow a regular exercise program.

Choose foods that are high in nutrition and moderate in calories. If you've heard this "balanced" and "moderate" stuff so often that you could recite it yourself, there's a reason for that: It's good for your health, and it works.

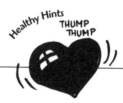

Healthy Hints
THUMP
THUMP

Pyramid Power

All calories are not created equal. A food choice can be a good source of nutrition or a source of empty calories. A good structure is the Food Guide Pyramid. If you need a reminder, bookmark The Food Guide Pyramid: A Guide to Daily Food Choices at http://www.nal.usda.gov:8001/py/pmap.htm. Also print out the pyramid and post it on your refrigerator.

Forget the impossible claims and hocus-pocus remedies. Here's the simple truth: Your weight is determined by the number of calories you take in versus the number of calories you use as energy, tempered by your metabolic rate. Some activities, such as sitting and reading this book, burn very few calories. Other activities, such as reading this book while you run on a treadmill, burn gobs of calories.

Calories from high-fat foods set up camp on your belly and thighs more easily than protein and complex carbohydrate calories, but whatever the source, if you consume more calories than you burn, you gain weight. It's science—there's just no way around it. Whether these extra calories come from cheeseburgers or fat-free cookies, if they're more than your body needs, they turn into stored body fat.

Fortunately, the opposite is also true. Burn more calories than you consume, and you whittle away your fat stores. You lose weight most successfully with a two-pronged attack: eating less and getting more active.

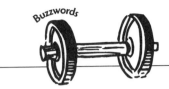

Buzzwords

Metabolic rate: The rate at which you burn calories. This varies from person to person, and is raised by physical activity and by amount of muscle mass.

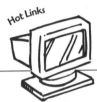

Hot Links

Winning by Losing: A Guide to Effective Weight Control

http://www.caloriecontrol.org/winweigh.html

The Calorie Control Council provides an excellent article discussing the truth about losing weight: "Successful weight control requires fewer calories and regular exercise, combined with healthy eating habits that can be maintained for life." (Can we stand all this good sense?) While you're at http://www.caloriecontrol.org/, you can find out how many calories are in that bag of chips you're holding by clicking Calorie Counter Calculator.

Junk Food: Eat It, Wear It

Although calories in/calories out (plus genetics—more about that later) basically determines our weight, it does matter whether these calories are coming from bananas or banana cream pie, from baked potatoes or potato chips. Food that is high in fat, high in calories, and low in nutrition is more apt to pile on the pounds than food your body requires for nutrition. Besides, you tend to eat higher quantities of high-fat, high-calorie foods than nutritious ones, taking in many more calories at a time than you realize.

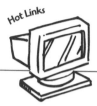

Food Finder

http://www.olen.com/food/

Want to know how much damage you did with that Double Bacon/Egg Burrito from Taco Bell? 480 calories (250 of them from fat), and one-fourth the fiber and ten times the cholesterol of a Burrito Supreme! The Food Finder site enables you to search by food and by fast-food restaurants (see Figure 13.1).

Figure 13.1

The Food Finder offers a searchable database of nutritional information for more than 1,000 fast-food items.

Move It or You Won't Lose It

When you make exercise a key part of your weight-loss program, you have an easier time losing weight and keeping it off than if you try to do it with diet alone. Exercise burns calories while you're active, and also raises your metabolic rate (the rate at which you burn calories) for hours later.

As if that weren't reason enough to get moving, the more muscle you gain, the faster your metabolic rate, even when you're at rest! That's because muscle requires more calories than fat. Each pound of muscle uses 30 to 50 calories a day just to sustain itself. A pound of fat uses only 2 to 3 calories per day! So, get active, including strength training for some attractive muscle, and that muscle will work away, chewing on your calories even while you're sprawled on the sofa watching *Judge Judy*.

Off Your Rocker

Here's a move Joan calls "Get Off Your Rocker" when she teaches it to her clients. Ready? Stand up. Sit down. Stand up. Sit down. Stand up. Repeat until you're tired or that slow Web page has loaded, whichever happens last. Advanced exercisers: Don't sit all the way down. When your cute little behind is almost on the chair, pop back up again. And again. And again.

So, if you skipped the exercise section of this book, go back now and read it very carefully—it's your ticket to weight-loss success.

Unrealistic Expectations

So, you've never looked like Cher. Even Cher has trouble looking like Cher and admits to extensive and expensive surgical aids. Let's face it, that slim, willowy look that lets you bare your navel with abandon belongs to teenagers who haven't reached their full growth yet, fitness fanatics who work out for hours every day, models who starve themselves, and a few genetically perfect individuals who defy all reason. The rest of us can improve our shape and size, but we can't reconfigure our body type.

If you want to know the body you inherited, look at the parent or grandparent you resemble the most (or who tells you, "I looked just like you when I was younger!"). Let's say, just for example, that it's Mom. Look at younger photos of Mom and see whether you can see the resemblance. Look at photos of her at her heaviest and slimmest.

Now look at Mom's activity level. If she's a sofa spud who lives on taco chips, then her body (sorry, Mom) reflects what yours will look like if you ignore all our good advice. If she's active and eats a healthy diet, there's your future if you do everything right.

Whatever your body type, you're bound to be happier if you aim for the weight at which you feel healthiest and most vigorous than to beat yourself up because you'll never be mistaken for Cindy Crawford or be able to wear Shania Twain's leopard-skin pants.

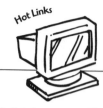

Hot Links

Weight Loss on FitnessLink

http://www.fitnesslink.com/weightloss/

FitnessLink has a fine collection of articles on different topics relating to weight loss. You'll learn how to figure out your caloric need for your ideal weight, whether your extra pounds are cause for concern, and secrets of people who were successful at losing weight. You can also calculate your BMI, and find quality-rated links to weight-loss sites.

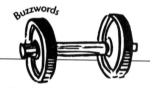

Buzzwords

BMI (Body Mass Index) : A ratio between weight and height that correlates to body fat and is considered a more accurate predictor of disease risk than scale weight.

Researching Weight Loss Online

The World Wide Web doesn't make pounds vanish, but it does get you on the right track to achieve that goal yourself. Your first need is information you can depend on. The following sites contain some quality resources.

Choosing a Safe and Successful Weight-Loss Program

http://www.niddk.nih.gov/health/nutrit/pubs/choose.htm

This article explains what to look for in a weight-loss program from the Weight-Control Informational Network of the National Institute of Diabetes and Digestive and Kidney Diseases of the National Institutes of Health. Following are the five basic requirements of a successful weight-loss program (you can learn much more by reading the article online):

1. Nutritionally safe and sound
2. Slow (one pound a week) and steady weight loss
3. Physician evaluation for more than 15- to 20-pound weight-loss goal
4. Plans for weight maintenance after the weight loss phase is over
5. Full disclosure of fees and additional items

Guidelines for Selecting a Weight-Loss & Maintenance Program

http://www.americanheart.org/Health/Risk_Factors/Overweight/Fad_Diets/
fadguide.html

Read these guidelines from the American Heart Association before choosing any weight-loss program. Besides guidelines, this online brochure lists the questions to consider before joining a program, and explains popular and ineffective weight-loss concepts, such as food combining and high-protein diets. You can also read articles from this site about other weight-loss topics.

Information About Losing Weight and Maintaining a Healthy Weight

http://vm.cfsan.fda.gov/~dms/wh-wght.html

This unadorned site from U.S. Food and Drug Administration, Center for Food Safety and Applied Nutrition, offers several articles on weight loss, such as "Weight-Loss Device Recalled," "Facts About Weight-Loss Products," "The New Food Label: Making It Easier to Shed Pounds," "Losing Weight Safely," and "Protecting Yourself from Health Fraud."

Evaluating Weight-Loss Web Sites by Using the PILOT Method

Remember the PILOT method we described in Chapter 3, "Junk or Jewel? Evaluating Web Site Content and Protecting Yourself"? Reread it now, or refresh your memory with the tear card. Here's how to apply it to weight-loss Web sites:

P Purpose   Look for a site that is set up to inform the public about safe and sensible ways to lose weight, not to sway you to a particular point of view or sell a product.

I Information   Is the information on the site based on sensible weight-loss guidelines that are endorsed by major health organizations, as are presented here? Or does the site veil the sale of a weight-loss product by using testimonials, vague descriptions, and too-good-to-be-true claims?

L Links   Quality Web sites offer links to other reputable, informational sites. They don't link to suspect sites or hold you captive.

O Originator   Pay little attention to sites run by individuals or companies that have a product to sell or an axe to grind. Pay no attention to testimonials—you can't trust them, you don't know what else the person was doing to lose weight, and you don't know how this approach will work for you.

T Timeliness   If the site is updated frequently, it reflects the current thinking of weight-loss experts.

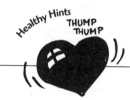

Commercial Weight-Loss Programs

We don't advocate weight-loss programs that supply prepackaged foods, because they don't teach you how to make food choices in the real world and they make you feel restricted, deprived, and ready to bail. Still, people join these programs. If you are sure that a prepackaged food program will help you, we caution you to explore it carefully before joining—and using the Internet can help. The following site is an example of how the Web can help you evaluate a weight-loss program before you spend your time and money on it.

Jenny Craig

```
http://www.jennycraig.com
```

Jenny Craig's site offers some good tips in its "Guide to Feeling Fit," and it details how its program works. Browsing through this site gives you a feel for the program and whether or not its menus and style might work for you. You can search for a center near you, or you can have your food delivered to your door via UPS if you live too far from a Jenny Craig center. Hmmm...food delivered via UPS—now that sounds appetizing! We recommend eating fresh foods that give you maximum nutrition and energy and help you learn how to follow a healthy diet that lasts a lifetime.

Sticking to It: Sites to Keep You Losing

You've decided what kinds of changes you want to make in your diet and lifestyle. Now don't you wish you had a helper, guide, dietitian, and menu advisor to guide you through the process step-by-step and help you stay on track? You do—online!

CyberDiet

```
http://www.cyberdiet.com/
```

This site is a terrific source for the good kind of diet information. Read interesting articles by registered dietitians on how you need to adapt your diet to the differing requirements of your age or the amount of weight you want to lose. CyberDiet enables you to assess your daily calorie and nutrient requirements with a personalized nutritional profile based on your needs and goals. Then check out the daily food planner, food facts, exercise tips, and recipe index, or talk to others about weight-loss issues in one of CyberDiet's 14 message boards.

Calorie Control Council

http://www.caloriecontrol.org

Some people like counting beats in a song, reps in a strength-training session, minutes until it's time to go home, so why not calories? We don't recommend counting every calorie, because it tends to make food even more of an obsession than it is already. But it's extremely useful to check the calorie count of suspect foods. For example, you really should know that 1/2 cup of chocolate mousse (when did you ever eat just 1/2 cup?) has 189 calories and 16 grams of fat. In contrast, 1/2 cup of chocolate soufflé has only 63 calories and 4 grams of fat. This site also offers news stories and articles concerning nutrition and weight loss.

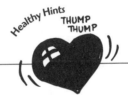

Healthy Hints THUMP THUMP

Drink and Grow Fat

Calorie for calorie, solid food fills you up more, and for longer, than drinks do, says Richard Mattes, professor of foods and nutrition at Purdue University. His 1998 research confirms a similar study he conducted in 1996: that when people drink alcohol or soda, they do not compensate for those extra calories by consuming less solid food. Soda consumption in the United States has nearly tripled since 1968, according to the National Soft Drink Association. Nationwide, four of the ten leading grocery items are beverages: soft drinks, juices, milk, beer. And, says a Purdue report, alcohol is the third highest single source of calories in this country: more than 5 percent of the total. All this liquid–dieting is a major reason why America's waistline has continuously expanded at the same time its overall fat consumption has decreased, Mattes said.

Nourish Net

http://www.nourishnet.com

This site offers weight-management support, including diet plans, recipes, healthy habits, exercise, and nutrition. Read a step-by-step plan for getting started, eating out, and more. Information is free, but if you want to join The Nourish Net Club, there's a fee (just like at noncyber weight-loss groups). The Club includes personal weight tracking and member support, including "food mentoring."

Shape Up America!

```
http://www.shapeup.org
```

Shape Up America!, C. Everett Koop's organization, is dedicated to "safe weight management, healthy eating, and physical fitness." First, find out how to calculate your BMI. Then go to the Fitness Center, take a fitness assessment test, and read about exercise and nutrition. There are menu plans based on the Food Guide Pyramid for 1,800, 2,000, and 2,500 calories. You can learn about weight-loss supplements, get healthy recipes, and figure out how many calories you burn in your normal activities each week.

The Least You Need to Know

➤ No gimmicky diet works as well as a nutritious lifelong eating plan that's moderate in calories and low in fat.

➤ Muscle can be your best weight-loss friend.

➤ Have realistic weight-loss expectations.

➤ Use the PILOT method to find reputable online weight-loss and nutrition sites for information and motivation.

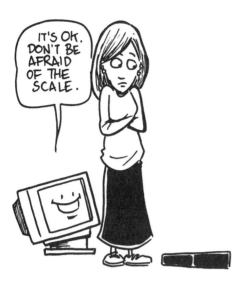

Chapter 14

Finding a Friend: Weight-Loss Support and Motivation Online

> ## In This Chapter
>
> ➤ Finding resources to help you stick to a weight-loss plan
>
> ➤ Exploring commercial support sites
>
> ➤ Locating friends online to support you in reaching your goals

You've got the information and you know the changes you have to make. But it can be a lonely world when you're trying to lose weight on your own. When it's midnight and you're this close to pillaging your kids' stash of Snickers bars, you can turn to support online to keep you on track. Whether you need a pep talk, a pity party, or a good friend with whom to share stories, you'll find it on the Internet.

Commercial Support Groups

Some people are more likely to succeed at weight loss by enrolling in a program or support group to keep them on task. Sitting at the computer with a pint of rocky road ice cream just inches from your fingertips is no substitute for actually showing up at a group meeting, but these sites at least let you know how to find a chapter near you.

Weight Watchers

```
http://www.weightwatchers.com/
```

Benvenuti nelle pagine di Weight Watchers! This is an international site, so just for fun, you can click on the flag of an intriguing country and read the introduction in a new language. Then you can get serious and search for a meeting in your city. "Weight Watchers maintains the global philosophy that healthful weight management involves a comprehensive program that includes a food plan, activity plan, and behavior modification provided in an environment of group support."

TOPS (Take Off Pounds Sensibly)

http://www.tops.org

"Offering a healthy, caring, and supportive approach to weight control, at an affordable price, has been our goal since 1948." TOPS has almost 275,000 members in 11,000 chapters throughout the world. No products, no hype, just fellowship through weekly meetings. You can find your closest meeting by entering your zip code or Canadian Postal Code.

Overeaters Anonymous

http://www.overeatersanonymous.org

OA is a community of people who support one another through the process of recovering from compulsive overeating with a 12-step program. "Our primary purpose is to abstain from compulsive overeating and to carry the message of recovery to those who still suffer." Learn about how OA works, read the 12 Steps and the Tools of Recovery, and then phone or email to find the closest meeting. No dues or fees.

Calf Shaper

Take a one-minute break from the computer. Stand on a phone book (the bigger, the better) with your heels hanging over the edge. Push up onto the balls of your feet for two seconds, hold in that position for two seconds, and then let yourself down again for four seconds. If you can't balance well enough to keep from careening off the phone book, lightly touch a wall or chair. Repeat for one minute, or until your calves are tired, whichever comes first. Advanced: Lift one leg slightly so you're doing the leg raises balancing on one leg at a time.

Online Support and Motivation

There's nothing like a buddy, or dozens of buddies, to help you stay on track and working toward your weight-loss goals. If you want to talk to a real person (or hundreds of them) but it's 2:00 a.m., or you're shy, or you're supposed to be working, or you've got diapers to change, the Internet provides a pipeline. Tools such as mailing lists, newsgroups, chat rooms, bulletin boards, and email pen pals give you the opportunity to discuss your goals, emotions, and successes with others who are going through the same experiences.

Mailing Lists

Weight-loss support mailing lists come in two forms:

➤ Lists that provide discussion of diet and weight-loss issues

➤ Lists that distribute newsletters, tips, or motivation for weight loss.

Using one of the mailing list search sites from Chapter 2, "What's Out There: The Many Faces of Online Health and Fitness Information," you can find mailing lists that discuss everything from general weight-loss issues to specific "fad" diets (do we have to remind you to avoid those?).

A good list should have a Web site that provides details about the list. Before joining, visit the list's Web site to find out how active the list is and the focus and topics of the discussion. We suggest the Fit and Trim Support Group. Share your struggles and successes with others on this list, which includes plenty of information on natural weight loss and exercise. To learn more about the list, go to `http://www.families-first.com/fitandtrim/`.

Newsgroups

Newsgroups are chancier than mailing lists, because anyone can access them and they are often the chosen tool for spammers who are looking to promote the latest too-good-to-be-true gimmick. You also have to be careful to weed through all the chatter about "fad" diets (the Zone and Atkins are recurring favorites—please review Chapter 13, "It's No Mystery: Losing Weight Safely and Effectively," and Chapter 15, "Promising the Moon: Beware of Fad Diets, Outrageous Claims, and Magic," if you're tempted). But aside from all that, you can often find extremely knowledgeable and supportive people who are willing to answer your questions, give you encouragement, and offer new ways to look at your weight-loss efforts. Try these: `alt.support.diet` and `sci.med.nutrition`.

Easy Ab Strengthener

Contract your abdominal muscles while you're sitting at the computer. Exhale and pull your abdominal muscles in firmly, as if you are buttoning a pair of jeans that are too tight (something that we're sure has never happened to you). Hold your abdominals in, breathing shallowly, for 6 to 10 seconds. Release the contraction and take a deep breath, and then contract again. Do this several times an hour.

Chat Rooms

A cyber room of strangers can quickly become friends because they understand and support your weight-loss goal. What could be better than connecting with others who want to help you, and whom you can help? Although there are several software programs out there that offer enhanced chat capabilities on the Internet, you don't *need* any fancy software to chat (go back to Chapter 2, and review the section on CyberFriends: Chat). Just find a Web site or chat room and start making friends!

If you subscribe to one of the online services (AOL, CompuServe, Prodigy), you'll find diet and weight-loss chat rooms by simply searching for the keywords "weight loss chat." Otherwise, you can find chat rooms on many weight-loss-related Web sites. Try the keywords "weight loss chat" in your favorite search engine, or start out with these two that we like:

➤ **Diet Talk**   http://www.diettalk.com/chat.htm
➤ **Weight Loss at About.com**   http://weightloss.about.com/mpchat.htm

Bulletin Boards

Bulletin boards, also known as forums, carry the same warnings as newsgroups: Beware of so-called experts giving advice, and scroll past posts concerning gimmicks and fads. But find a quality Web site with a bulletin board that is moderated, and you strike weight-loss-support gold.

Web bulletin boards are easy to use—you just go to the Web site and post your message. They typically have fewer people than newsgroups, letting you form a bond by joining a "community" of people who are looking to lose weight and support one another. A good bulletin board is hard to find—there are so many online, and few searches will find them all. Try Forum One, http://www.forumone.com, a search engine for forums. You can also seek out good weight-loss information sites; some have active bulletin boards which invite you to participate. One board we like is CyberDiet's Buddies Forum at http://www.cyberdiet.com/messages/dietbuddies/.

To evaluate a bulletin board, follow these steps:

➤ **Scroll through the postings and take note of the dates.** An active board should have at least a few postings per day.

➤ **Look over the subject lines of the postings.** They should be descriptive and supportive. If the subject lines are off-topic, abusive, or advertisement-driven, be wary of the board's content.

➤ **Read a few of the postings.** Do the people seem to know one another and respond kindly to questions, no matter how trivial? Is there a sense of community? Is there an absence of advertising for weight-loss scams and diet frauds?

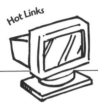

Hot Links

Richard Simmons

http://www.richardsimmons.com/

You can be part of the great motivator's in-group—just visit his Web site (see Figure 14.1), join his "club," and get personalized messages from Richard when you log in and by email. His site has a "Helpin' Board," where you can post or read questions and get help motivating yourself. Of course, he wants you to buy his videos and join his next cruise, but there's also a lot of free help, a daily motivational message, and live "auditoriums" with Richard.

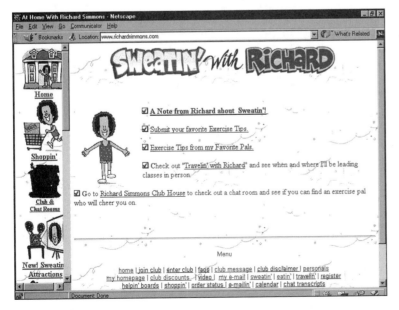

Figure 14.1

Richard Simmons' home on the Web motivates and supports your weight-loss efforts.

Email Pen Pals

Email has become the correspondence method of choice, with more than 90 million consumer emailboxes in the United States. Forrester Research predicts that nearly 50 percent of the U.S. population will communicate via email by the year 2001. How can you use this simple tool to help you achieve your weight-loss goals? Find some email pen pals!

With so many people using email these days, it's easy to find others who share your struggle and who will motivate and support you. Shelly Wistie, a fitness instructor at Gold's Gym in Olympia, WA, is living proof that email pen pals can make a difference in your life. Shelly found her friend, Edna, through FitnessLink's "Find a Friend for Weight Loss Support" at http://www.fitnesslink.com/news/friend.htm, and went from 290 to 175 pounds. Shelly writes:

"I have made the most incredible friend through 'Find a Friend for Weight-Loss Support!' I had posted on many boards regarding my struggle in my weight loss and my dream of becoming an aerobics instructor. The story begins—'you've got mail'— from Edna, an aerobics instructor in the LA area. She gave me such encouragement and praise for my accomplishments to date and said 'go for it.' At that time, I really didn't think I had what it took to be an aerobics instructor! I'd been doing aerobics since high school and after college had an injury, got married, got a 40-hour sit-at-your-desk job, and gained almost 150 pounds in four years. I had let myself go and really had no self-esteem left. But as I slowly took control of my life and got back into the fitness industry, Edna gave me courage and support. She actually typed up a 40-page study guide for a certification exam I had been studying for. Now that is a supportive friend! She sent me my first two aerobics tapes to start practicing, gave me ideas on choreography and just inspired me to teach. Amazing—someone I have never met could influence my life so much. I've seen talk shows and read articles about online romances—but there are so many other friendships and support groups online which are just amazing...I'm proof!"

Another excellent site for finding email pen pals is Diet Buddy, http://www.dietbuddynetwork.com (see Figure 14.2). If you're looking for online support, this is a great place to start. Here you can read through a huge list of dieters looking for buddies or post your own message. They offer a mailing list so you can get diet support delivered to your email box every morning. Also included are chats, bulletin boards, success stories, and links.

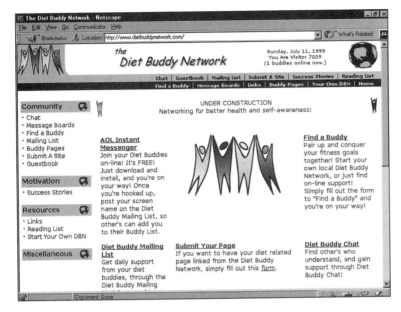

Figure 14.2

The Diet Buddy Web site helps you find weight-loss support and inspiration online.

The Least You Need to Know

➤ The Internet is a gold mine of weight-loss support.

➤ You can search the Internet for a commercial weight-loss support group or meeting in your area.

➤ People are willing to help you reach your weight-loss goals through online tools such as mailing lists, newsgroups, chat rooms, bulletin boards, and email pen pals.

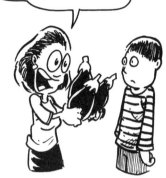

Chapter 15

Promising the Moon: Beware of Fad Diets, Outrageous Claims, and Magic

In This Chapter

➤ Recognizing the slimy weight-loss ploys

➤ Avoiding disreputable diets

➤ Evaluating weight-loss products

The World Wide Web teems with useful weight-loss information, useless weight-loss misinformation, and a dog pile of advertisers trying to sell you tomfoolery disguised as the answer to the body of your dreams. Joan did a search on "weight loss" on Infoseek—she got a list of 7,952,710 related Web sites. Sure, all these diets, programs, plans, gadgets, and schemes work—but they work for the seller, not necessarily for you. There are greedy scoundrels out there feeding on your desperation to lose weight, and they know that you'll buy anything that promises to answer your prayers. The sad truth is that most of these products and diets lighten only your wallet.

We won't embarrass you by asking how many of these schemes you've fallen prey to already. We're satisfied if you don't get taken in again. This chapter shows you how to recognize the warning signs that the weight-loss breakthrough of the millennium is really just another effort to bilk you out of your hard-earned cash.

Why Diet Is a Four-Letter Word

Thirty-four percent of adult Americans are overweight—an estimated 58 million. 50 million Americans will go on diets this year. Americans spend $30 billion a year on diet programs and products. Yet, with all this dieting going on, only about 5 percent

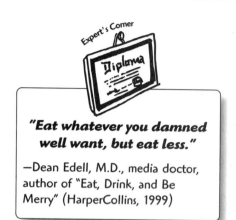

will keep the weight off long-term. We try diet after diet, but usually keep or regain the weight. So, why do we keep doing something that doesn't work?

You eat salads and skinned chicken breast for a couple of months, lose some pounds, go crazy with boredom, and return to the French fries and fat-oozing cheeseburgers. Then, you try one of the fad diets—cardboard and cabbage, let's say—and make yourself sick and irritable because of lack of nutrition. One of the problems with diets is that you're either on them or off them. The other problem is that they're rarely healthy. Those two points could make a book in themselves (*The Complete Idiot's Guide to Losing Weight* is a splendid example), but here it is in a nutshell: The real key is not to "diet," but to change the way you eat for the long haul.

Forget the trendy food combinations. Forget the high-protein diet disaster. (If it's so good, why does it come around and die again every decade, and why do almost all dietitians agree that it's unhealthy?) The only reason any of these diets seem to work in the beginning is that you're reducing calories (you can figure that out without sinking bucks into a diet plan) and often you're losing water weight.

What Do You Have to Lose?

People who are miserable about their weight are vulnerable to all sorts of scams and schemes. All scams take your money, but weight-loss scams take your dreams and your dignity. And sometimes they take your health. Weight-loss fraud bilks Americans out of an estimated $10 to $40 billion a year. (Why the wide range? How many of us report when we've been swindled by one of these frauds?)

Recognizing Quacky Diets and Weight-Loss Schemes

You've heard it a million times: "If it sounds too good to be true, it probably is." When you relate this to weight loss, you can safely delete the "probably."

You can spot a quacky diet or weight-loss scheme—online and offline—because it appeals to your emotions, not your reason. There's no mystery about how to lose weight. Increase your physical activity, decrease your calorie intake, make healthy food choices, avoid high-fat and high-calorie foods, and eat to fill physical, not emotional, hunger. Unless your genes fight you—and we'll talk about that later—that's how to lose weight. No "special, breakthrough ingredient." No "millions of satisfied customers." No "amazing results."

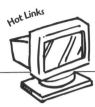

Hot Links

The Facts About Weight-Loss Products and Programs

http://vm.cfsan.fda.gov/~dms/wgtloss.html

This fact-filled online brochure is presented as a public service by the Federal Trade Commission, the Food and Drug Administration, and the National Association of Attorneys General. If you don't believe them, whom will you believe? They give you the scoop on what claims you shouldn't believe, with examples of weight-loss scams. "Appetite suppressing eyeglasses" and "magic weight-loss earrings," anyone?

Here's the bottom line. You can get good weight-loss information online from a government-sponsored site, a medical or dietetic organization (look for the ".gov" or ".org" in the URL), one of the reputable online health or nutrition magazines or newsletters, a credible and recognized weight-loss program such as Weight Watchers (http://www.weightwatchers.com), or a fitness site such as FitnessLink (http://www.fitnesslink.com). This information is always free. If you're asked to send money for a diet, plan, or product, tuck that credit card back into your wallet. A book or a cassette tape might be worth buying if you're satisfied with the credentials and expertise of the author, but there's no magic bullet to put in your weight-loss gun. Anyone who is trying to sell you a magic bullet knows that, and doesn't care about your weight, your self-esteem, your health, or anything but your money.

Spotting the Scams

Want to know if you should buy those slimming insoles, natural algae patches, or inch-zapping, fat-blocking pills? Here's where you can find more information on your weight-loss gimmick of choice. Better still, use these resources to help you protect your dough.

The Latest Weight-Loss Gimmicks

http://www.weight.com/gimmick.html

Metabolic stimulants, weight-loss ear patches, slimming soaps, magnets! Michael D. Myers, M.D., lists current gimmicks and answers questions about whether they work.

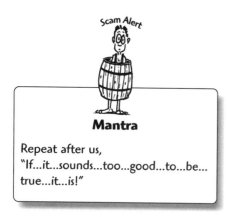

Mantra

Repeat after us,
"If...it...sounds...too...good...to...be...
true...it...is!"

Dr. Myers is a physician in Los Alamitos, California, who treats obesity and eating disorders.

Quackwatch

http://www.quackwatch.com/

Go to the enormous list of "Questionable Products, Services, and Theories" and scroll to "Weight Control Gimmicks and Frauds." Here you find this year's "Slim Chance Awards" for weight-loss schemes by Frances M. Berg, M.S., editor of *Healthy Weight Journal*. Links to past years' awards are also here. If you'd rather type than scroll, you can get there directly: http://www.quackwatch.com/01QuackeryRelatedTopics/PhonyAds/slim/9 9.html.

Fat City

http://www.dietfraud.com/file-diet-complaints.html

Have you been scammed by a weight-loss scheme? Are you getting weight-loss emails beyond your endurance? You have recourse! This page explains how to complain about diet and weight-loss fraud, what agency to contact for which kind of problem, from weight-loss fraud to junk emails, with links to the agencies' sites. This page is part of the Fat City Web site (http://www.dietfraud.com), which is your diet and weight-loss fraud headquarters from Dr. Terry Polevoy, Waterloo, Ontario, Canada. Learn the truth about fraudulent weight-loss products, including how to take legal action.

Two Guys with a Placebo

Ken and Ron Brown, two Boomer-aged brothers from California, were looking for a way to make some cash by selling something on the Internet. They looked at what was raking in the bucks in the health area—mostly gimmicks for weight loss, sexual problems, and antiaging. So they decided, hey, instead of selling a junk product that claims to do the impossible and pretending it works, let's spoof junk products and advertise honestly a novelty product that doesn't work but is cleverly advertised!

So, Ken and Ron invented three products, which you can check out at http://members.aol.com/krbsr/page3.html: Na-tur-L for Men (improves "tired penis syndrome"—just rub it on, and rub, and rub), Na-tur-L for Women ("the natural treatment for wrinkled and sagging breasts"), and our favorite, Liquid Fat! "Eliminate strenuous exercise, fad diets! Just add a capful of Liquid Fat to your bath water and bathe your fat away!!" the ad screams. The amount of weight you lose, of course, depends on how often you bathe! Ken and Ron added this pseudoscientific (that means fake science, garbage, worthless) explanation (see Figure 15.1):

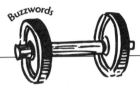
Buzzwords

Placebo: A drug or other preparation that has no real medicinal effect but is given for its psychological effect on the patient.

Placebo effect: This occurs when patients who believe a substance will work often get better even when their recovery has nothing to do with what the substance contains.

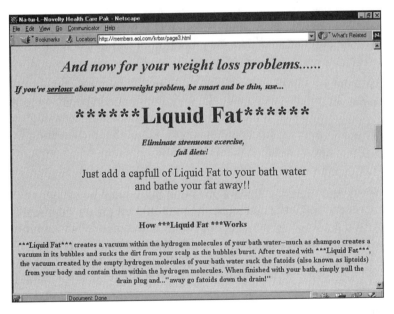

Figure 15.1

Even though Ken and Ron Brown proudly proclaimed their product to be a placebo, people started putting in real orders for "Liquid Fat."

Ken and Ron had no intention to rip people off. "I wanted my product to look so real, people will look at it and think about buying it—then realize it's all a joke, have a laugh—and buy it anyway, so they can show their friends and everybody can laugh," explains Ken. "And at the same time, maybe they will have learned something about buying junk products just because the label or the advertising says it works."

Their good intentions backfired, though. Even though they proudly proclaimed their product to be a placebo, people started ordering it for real! One weight-loss hopeful ordered six bottles of Liquid Fat. Ken and Ron started replying to their customers that they couldn't sell them the product unless they realized that it was a novelty item and would not really work—after which most canceled their orders.

The point to this long story is this: There are a lot of worthless products out there claiming to provide the answer to your dreams. A minuscule percentage of those sellers are as honest as Ken and Ron. Don't fall for it! If any of these products really worked, don't you think they'd be front-page news instead of hidden away on a stranger's Web site? If it sounds too good to be true, it is!

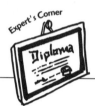

"Don't get your information from the same source where you buy your product. Get it from health and fitness experts who are licensed, highly qualified, and recommended by other highly qualified and licensed professionals within the health and fitness fields."

—Ken Brown, who learned how gullible people are when they ordered his fake products from his Internet ad

Diet Books

There are go-on-a-diet books and there are change-your-diet books. Go-on-a-diet books are most likely to become bestsellers, because they sell dreams rather than reality. Do something, anything, for three weeks or six weeks or 180 days, and you might or might not lose some weight, but it's short term. Ask any yo-yo dieter how much weight he or she has lost, and you'll be surprised at the number of pounds and the number of times this has happened. Losing weight is easy—keeping it off is the tricky part.

Keeping it off is no mystery, either. If you ate certain amounts of certain foods and gained weight, you can't do something different for a while, return to the old way of eating, and hope to keep the weight off. Look at Oprah Winfrey, for goodness sake. She went on a very low-calorie, impossible diet, wheeled a wagon of fat onto the TV stage to gloat about her weight loss, and a year later was wearing that fat on her body again. It wasn't until she started a sensible (don't we hate that word?) program of moderate calorie, low-fat eating plus exercise that she lost the old weight and could maintain the new weight.

There are excellent books that teach you how to do that—such as *The Complete Idiot's Guide to Losing Weight*, any of Dean Ornish's books, and Joan Price's *The Honest Truth About Losing Weight and Keeping It Off* (available from 1-888-BFITTER). But realize these are change-your-diet books, changes you make for life, not just for the class reunion.

Junk-Mail Crumple

Each time you get a piece of weight-loss scam junk mail, don't just toss it—crumple it first. Open the envelope and pull out the letter (don't read it!). Hold it with one hand. Start at one corner and crumple it into your palm, bit by bit, until it's one tight ball. Squeeze it a few times, and then drop it into the recycling container. Grab another junk letter with your other hand, and repeat. This strengthens your forearm, relieves wrist tension from overuse at the keyboard, and gives your junk mail some purpose during its very brief time in your life.

Read Before You Buy: Reviews, Excerpts Online

The online booksellers such as Amazon.com and Barnesandnoble.com not only provide an easy way to order books, but a fine source of information about books. You can read reviews, reader comments, and interviews with the author, and learn a lot before you buy. It's easy to separate the change-your-diet books from the go-on-a-diet books by reading about the book first.

Some publishers and authors have their own Web sites. For example, you can see a listing of chapters from Joan's book, *Joan Price Says, Yes, You CAN Get in Shape!* (it's not a diet book, but shows you how exercise is essential for getting you to your goals, and, hey, she'll take all the publicity she can get) at http://www.fitnesslink.com/joanprice/#book (see Figure 15.2), and you can read excerpts and other articles by scrolling up from there.

The Truth About Best-Selling Diet Books

If any of the best-selling diet books really helped us accomplish our goals, why would we need a pile of new ones every January (New Year's Resolutions) and April (countdown to bathing suits)? If the book you're considering promotes a radical, temporary change, or a change that doctors and dietitians refute, don't add it to your collection. (We know you have a collection!)

159

Figure 15.2

Joan's Web site offers excerpts and a listing of chapters from her book, Joan Price Says, Yes, You CAN Get in Shape!

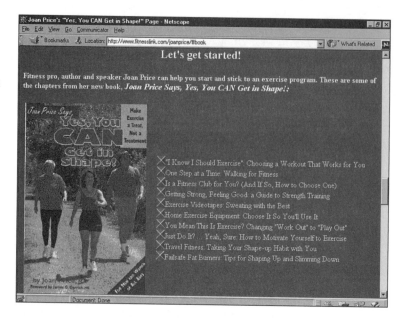

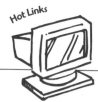

"How to Identify Weight-Loss Fraud"

`http://www.healthyweightnetwork.com/fraud.htm`

This is an online brochure by Frances M. Berg, national coordinator of the Task Force on Weight Loss Abuse of the National Council Against Health Fraud, editor of *Healthy Weight Journal*, and licensed nutritionist. She presents 24 guidelines for identifying a quack weight-loss site. She includes types of products considered fraudulent and how to report it if you do get scammed.

Weight-Loss Red Flags

Most weight-loss frauds are easy to spot after you know the signs. As we said previously, if someone wants money for a product or a plan, that red flag should be waving like a sheet in a tornado. Here are some claims that should send you running in the other direction, wallet tucked tightly away.

If you read Chapter 3, "Junk or Jewel: Evaluating Web Site Content and Protecting Yourself," you know to be wary of testimonials (including photos, and/or undocumented case histories), pseudoscientific or misused medical terms, references to studies without specific citations, and claims that the product treats a whole slew of conditions. Other dead giveaways are the following claims that online weight-loss schemes adore overusing.

"Burns Fat"

Nothing burns fat except exercising off excess calories. If you take in X calories and use up X + 100 calories, those extra 100 have to come from somewhere, so they come from your fat stores. No product does this for you. The only way to make it work is by just eating less and moving more.

"Gets Rid of Cellulite"

Cellulite is just a fancy French name for body fat. Yeah, it has a different appearance—sort of like cottage cheese under the skin. That's because the skin is thin in those areas, and the fat puckers up at you. You get rid of cellulite the same way you get rid of any other kind of body fat. No magic, sorry!

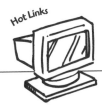

Hot Links

Quackwatch: Cellulite

http://www.quackwatch.com/01QuackeryRelatedTopics/cellulite.html

(If that's too much typing, go to http://www.quackwatch.com/ and scroll until you see Cellulite Removers.)

Stephen Barrett, M.D., nails cellulite ads with a clear, scientific explanation of what cellulite is (and isn't), with descriptions and evaluations of dozens of products that don't work. If you're in danger of being swayed by the ads, read this article first! It links to some of the bunko ads: body wraps, massagers, herbal products (with a long analysis of the fad of the moment, Cellasene), and a cream that claims to be "liposuction in a jar." (We refuse to give you the URL of that one—you'll find it *after* you read Dr. Barrett's article!)

"Without Diet or Exercise"

You can't lose weight without changing your diet and/or exercise habits. Period. Calories in, calories out, remember? If you keep eating the kind or amount of food that piled on the pounds in the first place, and your exercise is limited to the remote control boogie, any pill, lotion, gadget, or treatment that you can buy online reduces only your checking account.

Bozo Buzzwords: Magic, Secret, Easy, Effortless, Fast, Guaranteed, and Permanent

These buzzwords play on your dreams, not your reason. They're designed to get your hopes up and give you some sense of reassurance. Here they are, one by one:

➤ **Magic** There's no magic. If there were, we'd all have heard about it by now, and there would be no reason that a third of the population is overweight.

➤ **Secret** Excuse me, but why would an honest-to-goodness weight-loss discovery be kept secret? Get real!

➤ **Easy/Effortless** The truth is, it does take effort to watch your food and increase your exercise level. You wish it could be easy and effortless, but it just isn't.

➤ **Fast** Any diet or product that promises you'll lose a pound a day or anything over a pound or two a week is yanking your chain. You can lose more water than that, but not more body fat.

➤ **Guaranteed** A guarantee is as good as the company that stands behind it. Most people are too embarrassed to ask for their money back. Those who do are often ignored, or the company and Web site disappear (now there's permanent for you!), or there never was a company in the first place, just some greedy guy or gal cashing checks as quickly as possible.

➤ **Permanent** Dream on, honey. How could weight loss be permanent when you eat every day?

So, surf on to the next site when you see any of these words advertising a weight-loss product—or, for that matter, any health product. And if you find a site using all or most of these words—and any we haven't thought of—email the URL to Joan at jprice@sonic.net. We're collecting them for the next edition of this book!

162

Scam Test

Okay, here's a test to see how well you read this chapter. Go to the NordiCaLite Web site at http://www.ari.net/nordicalite (see Figure 15.3).

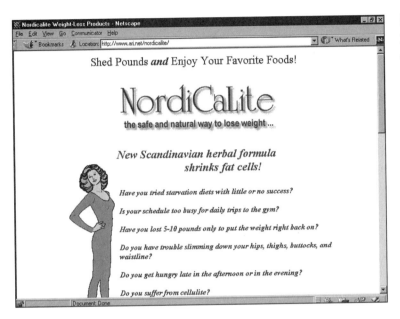

Figure 15.3

NordiCaLite flunks the scam test!

Sounds convincing, doesn't it? Who wouldn't want to "shrink fat cells" without rabbit food, exercise, hunger, pills, diet meals, or doctor visits!

By the way, what are they selling? Ah yes, we found it: "essence of Malmos—a unique blend of all-natural herbs derived from the evergreen forests of Scandinavia." Uh huh!

How many red flags, buzzwords, and other scam indicators can you find? Read all the way to the end of the page, because we don't want you to miss the "scientific" explanation of how the product works ("molecular isomers…this concentrated extract burns fat by encouraging isotonic thermogenesis…") and the impressive credentials of its inventor.

Ready for a surprise! This isn't even a real ad. And it's not a real product. No, we didn't make it up. The Federal Trade Commission was nice enough to put up the site to save you from yourself—although you don't learn that until you click **more** and then **SAVE EVEN MORE!** to get to page 3. Their aim: "to raise awareness about the false and deceptive advertising claims made by many so-called 'weight-loss' products."

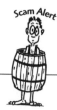

Gizmos and Gadgets

There is no device that will help you lose weight—other than a catapult that pulls you away from the table, stuffs your feet into your walking shoes, and propels you out the door. (Hey! Inventors, get in touch!) Phony weight-loss devices might be merely ineffective or downright destructive, especially to your pocketbook. Forget it.

The Least You Need to Know

➤ You can get valuable information about weight loss online.

➤ There are no shortcuts to losing weight, but there are plenty of scummy sites that will try to convince you otherwise.

➤ Unscrupulous peddlers give themselves away with warning signs, claims, and buzzwords that you can learn to recognize.

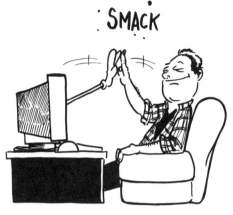

SMACK

Chapter 16

Accept It: Accepting Your Body and Your Weight

In This Chapter

➤ Understanding how your weight might be influenced by your genes

➤ Appreciating how to be healthy whatever your size

➤ Learning to accept your body as it is

Many people cannot lose weight no matter what they do, and the cost is monstrous not only in money ($30 billion to $50 billion yearly), but also in feelings of failure, guilt, anger and self-loathing. That's too big a price to pay. This chapter helps you get off the diet roller coaster and start to live your life fully, whatever your weight.

You Can Change Your Diet, but Not Your Genes

Nature, nurture, or choice? Although we've said that losing weight depends on taking in fewer calories and expending more calories through physical activity, there are people whose genes seem to preset their body weight, and neither dieting nor exercise seems to change it much. There's a theory that a body has a weight set point —a range it returns to as natural. Within that range, we can lose or gain weight, but we probably can't push ourselves out of that range. We can override it temporarily with heroic measures, but as soon as we relax our efforts, it zooms back to its comfortable range. So, if you renounce midnight snacks and your mother's fried chicken and you still can't lose weight, your genes (not jeans) might be responsible. In a nutshell, heredity might be more important than your lifestyle choices.

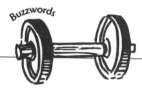

Buzzwords

Set point: Theoretically, a mechanism that sets your weight range, similar to a thermostat. You carry a certain amount of weight that your genes determine is right for your body. When your weight goes lower than your set point, your metabolism slows down so you gain the weight back.

This is a roundabout way of telling you that if you haven't been successful at losing weight and keeping it off even when you've done everything the way we recommended in Chapter 13, "It's No Mystery: Losing Weight Safely and Effectively," stop punishing yourself. It's not your fault. The good news is that people who are so-called overweight but fit (they exercise, don't smoke, and make good food choices) are often healthier than people who are slim but unfit.

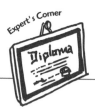

Expert's Corner

"At the height of my body shame and self-hatred in my twenties, a counselor told me: 'You'll never learn to love yourself until you learn to love your body.' At the time, I thought she was nuts. Couldn't she see how fat my thighs were, for heaven's sake? But, of course, she was right. No matter how long it takes, women who finally 'get it'—that we deserve to have a good life regardless of our size—are much more likely to gently and lovingly care for ourselves, and be healthier as a result. So, dance, play, rest, relax, eat, and enjoy life just as you are. Enjoy your body. It's the best home you'll ever have."

—Pat Lyons, RN MA, co-author of *Great Shape: The First Fitness Guide for Large Women* (Bull Pub., 1990); Director, Connections Women's Health Consulting Network, Oakland, CA

How to Tell Whether You're Genetically Heavy

We have no problem accepting that some people are naturally slim, no matter how much they eat. So, why is it so difficult to accept that some people are naturally heavy, no matter how little they eat? If we feel like placing blame, we can slam the media, or the snooty attitudes of thin people, or the glut of diet books and diet plans that really want a bite out of the billions spent on weight loss each year, or the fashion industry for not making flattering swimsuits, or trendy boutiques for not carrying plus sizes.

The fact is that some people gain weight because they eat too much, and others are genetically disposed to a higher weight and can't do a darn thing about it. To tell whether your genes are responsible, ask yourself these questions:

➤ What did you weigh as an adult during long periods when you were neither dieting nor overeating? (If you can't think of a time you were neither dieting nor overeating, we recommend you try it!)

➤ Is there a certain weight to which you gravitate, whatever you do?

➤ Do you have great difficulty losing weight during weight-loss efforts, even when you do everything right?

➤ When you lose weight, do you regain it quickly and end up at the weight you were before you lost weight?

Do you see a pattern here?

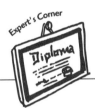

"Since many people cannot lose much weight no matter how hard they try, and promptly regain whatever they do lose, the vast amounts of money spent on diet clubs, special foods, and over-the-counter remedies, estimated to be on the order of $30 billion to $50 billion yearly, is wasted."

—from "Losing Weight—An Ill-Fated New Year's Resolution," editorial by Jerome P. Kassirer, M.D., and Marcia Angell, M.D., in *The New England Journal of Medicine*, January 1, 1998, Vol. 338, No. 1 (You can read this editorial online at http://www.nejm.org/content/1998/0338/0001/0052.asp.)

What You Can or Can't Do About It

What you can do is live the healthiest lifestyle—eat a variety of nutritious foods, avoid junk food, quit smoking, reduce stress, and engage in regular exercise or leisure physical activities that you enjoy. This keeps your body healthy and lively, decreasing your risk of lifestyle-related diseases.

What you can't do is force your body into a size that isn't natural for it. What you shouldn't do is drive yourself crazy because of it. Studies are finding that it's healthier to be heavy and fit than thin and unfit.

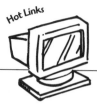

Hot Links

"Is Giving Up on Dieting Giving Up on Yourself?"

http://www.radiancemagazine.com/giving_up_on.html

For her Ph.D. research, Debby Burgard surveyed women who weighed over 200 pounds about issues related to their weight and attitudes about it, including their weight history, body image, dieting, beliefs about control over weight, social supports, day-to-day life as a large woman, and feelings about the acceptability of their weight. Over 100 women responded; average weight: 287 pounds; average number of attempts to lose weight: 40. Their beliefs will surprise you if you're convinced that you have to be slim to accept yourself. Read Burgard's article in *Radiance* magazine online.

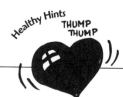

Healthy Hints

THUMP
THUMP

Is Your Weight-Loss Goal Self-Destructive?

➤ The average North American woman wears size 14.

➤ A typical model weighs less than 75 percent of an average woman's weight. This used to be 92 percent.

➤ More than 11 million North American females suffer from eating disorders.

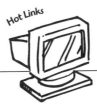

Hot Links

But I'm So Fat!

Fifty percent of adolescents are trying to lose weight. Fifty percent of fourth graders have dieted. This fixation on weight loss can lead to an eating disorder, such as anorexia nervosa, bulimia, or obsessive overeating. The following sites can help you recognize and understand eating disorders, and help someone who has one.

Eating Disorders Awareness and Prevention, Inc.

```
http://members.aol.com/edapinc/
```

This national nonprofit organization is dedicated to increasing the awareness and prevention of eating disorders, with programs and an instructive Web site. EDAP aims to educate people about eating disorders and eliminate the 3 Ds: "body dissatisfaction, dieting behavior, and drive for thinness." There are articles for parents, teens, kids, and friends.

The Something Fishy Web Site on Eating Disorders

```
http://www.something-fishy.org/
```

Amy, a member of the Something Fishy band, had anorexia. As she and her husband learned more about the disorder and how to cope with it, they started accumulating information for this Web site. It has grown into a large, informative site about all types of eating disorders, with a warm and personal touch. "If we can continue to come together with support and hope, I have faith there can be life after an eating disorder," writes Amy.

Self-Acceptance: Start Here

The Internet opens up a brave new world of sites, online magazines, role models, and support groups to help you accept yourself at any weight. The following resources are great starting points.

Radiance: The Magazine for Large Women

```
http://www.radiancemagazine.com
```

Radiance, the magazine "for women all sizes of large," is now online as well as on the newsstands (see Figure 16.1). Warm, sassy, and educational, *Radiance* covers stories that large women want to read. Each issue has an in-depth interview with a plus-size celebrity—such as Rosie O'Donnell and Camryn "this is for all the fat girls!" Manheim—and articles on health, media, fashion, and politics. Absolutely no diets. "We celebrate women all sizes of large, of all ages, lifestyles, and ethnicities. *Radiance* helps inspire its readers to live proud, full, active lives, now, with self-love and self-respect."

Figure 16.1

Radiance Magazine celebrates women of all sizes.

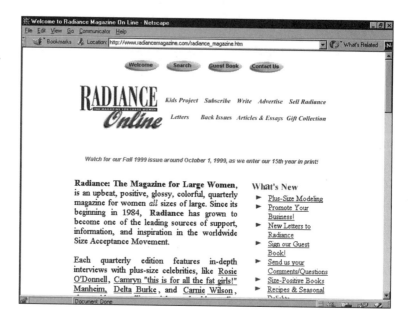

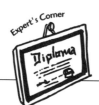

"Our bodies are beautiful, whatever their size or shape. You have every right to the pleasures and joys available to you in your life now. There is abundant support available to women of size—find it and use it!"

—Alice Ansfield, publisher and editor, *Radiance: The Magazine for Large Women*, www.radiancemagazine.com, Oakland, CA

Body Positive

http://www.bodypositive.com/

"Body Positive looks at ways we can feel good in the bodies we have." This site is about accepting yourself, being healthy, and enjoying your life, whatever your weight, by Debby Burgard, Ph.D., psychologist and co-author of *Great Shape: The First Fitness Guide for Large Women*. "Body Positive explores taking up occupancy inside your own skin, rather than living above the chin until you're thin. It is a set of ideas that may help you find greater well-being in the body you have."

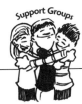

Support Groups

The Zoftig Zone Mailing List

http://www.eskimo.com/~leiba/zz/

A mailing list "created for people of size, their friends, and allies," the Zoftig Zone offers support and friendship, while promoting "tolerance, understanding, and insight" for overweight people.

Healthy Weight

http://www.healthyweightnetwork.com

Healthy Weight Network, including *Healthy Weight Journal*, aims to provide a link between research and practical application in weight and eating issues, edited by Frances M. Berg, M.S., a licensed nutritionist, family wellness specialist, and adjunct professor at the University of North Dakota School of Medicine. You're able to read news briefs and editorials about weight and health issues, such as the myths about dieting. "Recognizing that weight is an easily exploitable health and social concern, we are further committed to exposing deception, reshaping detrimental social attitudes, and promoting good health at any size. Our mission is to be a voice of integrity and insight in a field that has been much abused and neglected."

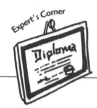

"For many years, I taught a class called 'We Dance—Exclusively for Women over 200 Pounds.' At the same time, I ran an inpatient program for women with eating disorders. I was working with the healthiest fat women in my dance classes and the sickest thin women in the hospital! It became very clear to me that health was not automatically linked to thinness. I couldn't ask a fat woman to embrace a diet mentality if that's what I thought was partly responsible for ruining the lives of my eating disordered patients."

—Debby Burgard, Ph.D., psychologist and co-author of *Great Shape: The First Fitness Guide for Large Women* (Bull Pub., 1990). Read more about it at http://www.bodypositive.com.

The Least You Need to Know

➤ Some people seem to be genetically programmed to have higher body weights.

➤ You can get fitter and healthier even if you don't lose weight.

➤ Self-acceptance is healthier physically and psychologically than obsessing about losing weight.

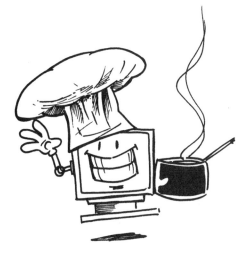

Chapter 17

Cooking Up a Storm: Healthy Cooking Tips and Recipes Online

In This Chapter

➤ Finding healthy recipes and recipe conversions online

➤ Understanding food terms and ingredients

➤ Turning your kitchen and refrigerator into a support system for maintaining a healthy lifestyle

Millions of recipes! Novel ways to spice up your tried and true recipes! Healthy cooking has never been easier—thanks to your special kitchen helper, the Internet. Shannon uses the Web on a regular basis to discover unique recipes that make her husband ask for seconds. She also finds recipes for homemade baby food to make her son gurgle with pleasure!

Ingredients for Healthy Cooking

The Internet can also be your healthy-cooking instructor. Discover which ingredients are too high in sugar, salt, or fat, and how to substitute healthier ones. Get tips for converting a familiar recipe to a more nutritious, lower-fat version. Maybe you see recipes in cookbooks, but don't have the ingredients called for, don't know where to find them, or don't even know what they are! You can learn almost anything about food and recipes using the Internet.

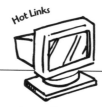

Epicurious Food Dictionary

http://www.epicurious.com/run/fooddictionary/home

What exactly does "al dente" mean? What is miso and why should we make soup with it? "Search our dictionary of more than 4,000 food terms and you'll never have to eat your words," promises Epicurious. Besides having a food dictionary, Epicurious has a wine dictionary and tons of food-related information.

The Healthy Refrigerator

One of the first steps you need to take toward cooking—and living—healthy is to clean the bad stuff out the fridge and cabinets and make room for some healthy essentials.

For tips on giving your refrigerator a healthy makeover, check out the Healthy Refrigerator site at http://www.healthyfridge.org/tips.html (see Figure 17.1).

This site offers some great tips for a heart-healthy refrigerator, such as hiding desserts in the crisper, away from view. This one works well for Shannon—she often forgets she bought that cheesecake in a moment of weakness! According to this site, Americans on average waste about $10 a week on produce that spoils—don't let that happen to you with the Healthy Refrigerator's tips for serving and storing produce.

The Fresher, the Better

Your next step to cooking up a healthy storm is to use fresh ingredients. Did you know that spices can go bad? Or that canned fruits and veggies usually have lots of additives and extra sodium? And those frozen entrée dinners—preservatives galore! For healthier cooking, spend more time in the produce section of your supermarket, and less time in the frozen food section.

Great Substitutions

So, you want to eat healthy, but your favorite recipes are from Grandma's Meat, Potatoes, and Gravy cookbook? Try the Cook's Thesaurus at http://www.switcheroo.com. This site offers thousands of low-fat and low-calorie ingredient substitutions. For example, you can substitute yogurt for mayonnaise in chicken and tuna salads, and substitute ground turkey for ground beef in any recipe. Also available are cheaper substitutes for chefs on a budget, and creative replacements for ethnic ingredients that you might not be able to find in your local supermarket.

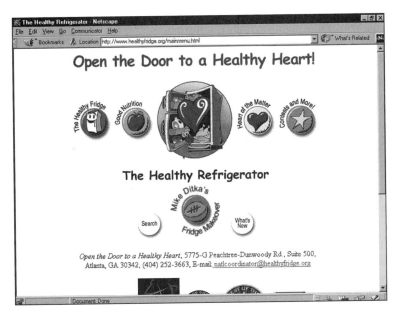

Figure 17.1

The Healthy Refrigerator Web site helps you "open the door to a healthy heart."

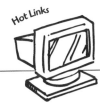

Hot Links

Picking Your Produce

`http://www.5aday.com`

"Only 27% of women and 19% of men report eating the recommended five servings of fruits and vegetables every day." This site offers useful information on sneaking those five servings of fruits and veggies into your diet. The recipe section discusses picking and storing produce and offers some great recipes. Be sure to explore the rest of the site—especially the links area, which provides information on nutrition content, health benefits, and links to other fruit and vegetable Web sites.

Expanding Your Mealtime Repertoire Using the Web

Are you tired of eating the same thing week after week? Does your family expect spaghetti on Mondays, chicken and rice on Wednesdays, and pizza on Fridays? Spice up your meals and expand your cooking repertoire by doing a little research on the Internet.

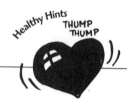

Healthy Hints

THUMP THUMP

Five Easy Ways to Prepare Healthier Meals

Eating healthier doesn't mean you have to sacrifice taste or texture. Give these tips a try!

➤ **Microwave**   Vegetables cook in little or no water, so they retain maximum flavor, color, and nutrients. Microwaving also cuts cooking times.

➤ **Steam**   Also done with the "lid on," most vegetables steam in minutes. Cook in a covered saucepan, in a colander or steamer basket, over a small amount of boiling water. The steaming liquid can be saved for soups and stews.

➤ **Stir-Fry**   It's really not "frying" at all. This technique requires very little oil. Cut foods into small, uniform pieces and toss constantly in a very hot skillet. Foods cook quickly and stay bright and crisp.

➤ **Stock Up on Broth**   Canned chicken or vegetable broth is good to keep on hand. Sometimes just the vegetables' natural juices are enough to keep them moist while cooking, but usually a little extra liquid is needed, especially with firmer vegetables. Plain water is okay, too, but the broth adds extra flavor. If you're trying to cut down on salt, look for reduced sodium broth.

—Courtesy of Wegmans Food Stores, http://www.wegmans.com

Learning More About Food

When you start following food-related links on the Web, you can find good info and bad info. All of the warnings about the safety of food might make you paranoid—you might be tempted to give up restaurants and buy food only directly from an organic farm. Don't let yourself get too crazed. Use your own judgment and, of course, the PILOT method, when looking at this type of site.

The National Food Safety Database, `http://www.foodsafety.org`, can help you sort out food safety issues with its many articles, tips, and links.

On the positive side, you can find out everything about every food in existence on the Internet. For example, the National Pasta Association's Web site, `http://www.ilovepasta.org/`, offers recipes, nutritional information, and a cool guide to pasta shapes which tells you the type of recipe or sauce for each shape of pasta (see Figure 17.2).

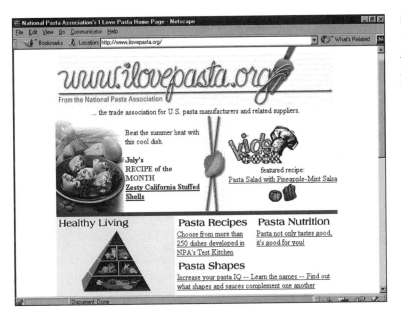

Figure 17.2

The National Pasta Association Web site gives you the lowdown on everything pasta.

Learning More About Shopping

Whether you consider shopping for food a joy or a chore, you could probably use some guidance on how to choose healthier fare. As already mentioned, spend lots of time in the produce section and stock up on fresh fruits and veggies. Be adventurous and buy a food you've never tried before. Then search the Web for the food you're considering, to find recipes from world-renowned chefs and someone's Aunt Betsy, restaurant reviews, and preparation tips.

Like shopping at home? For the ultimate convenience (or just for fun), check out NetGrocer, `http://www.netgrocer.com`, the online supermarket that delivers your order right to your door!

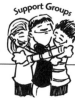

Sharing Your Recipe Secrets

Mailing lists and newsgroups are other wonderful places to swap cooking tips and recipes with others who share your passion. You can find groups that specialize in a particular type of cooking, have a more general dialog. Here are a few to check out:

➤ `rec.food.cooking`

➤ `alt.food.low-fat`

➤ Cook, `http://www.onelist.com/subscribe.cgi/cook`

➤ Favorite Recipes, `http://members.tripod.com/~Beckerbuns/weekly.html`

Cooking for Special Interests

Whatever your cooking (or eating) interests might be, you're sure to find plenty of recipes on the Internet.

Vegetarian

`http://www.vegsource.org`

VegSource has more than 5,000 vegetarian recipes in its directory—not to mention tons of other useful information for veggies.

Diabetes

`http://soar.berkeley.edu/recipes/diabetic`

The Searchable Online Archive of Recipes (SOAR) has a section devoted exclusively to diabetics.

Low-Fat and Fat-Free

`http://www.fatfree.com`

The Low-Fat Vegetarian Recipe Archive has more than 2,500 fat-free and low-fat vegetarian recipes.

Ethnic and Traditional

http://www.usgennet.org/~alhnfood/ethnic.html

This page includes an informative list of links to sites that offer ethnic recipes. Try your hand at cooking Cornish Pasties, Creole and Cajun recipes, traditional Jewish food, Tex-Mex, Maryland seafood, and more!

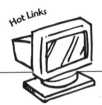

Hot Links

Online Cookbooks

Finding cookbooks online is almost as easy as finding recipes! In addition to the sites we recommend here, you can also check out bookseller giants Amazon.com (http://www.amazon.com) and Barnes and Noble (http://www.barnesandnoble.com) for cookbook reviews and easy online ordering. Both sites let you browse by category (in this case, "cooking").

CookeryBooks http://www.cookerybooks.com

CookeryBooks is an excellent site that enables you to search for cookbooks by author, title, category, or cuisine country. Each book listing provides publisher's description, and many listings also have reviews and sample recipes from the book.

Books-for-Cooks http://www.booksforcooks.com

"Let your imagination go at Books—for-Cooks.com and find the perfect cookbook for your taste!" More than 8,000 cookbooks, organized into categories.

StarChefs http://starchefs.com/Cookbooks/Picks.html

Read a list of best-selling cookbooks, as well as the StarChefs Staff Picks. Then, you can move on to an alphabetical list of cookbook reviews.

Kitchen Lunge

Here's an exercise that strengthens and defines your thighs and buttocks while you're waiting for the water to boil. Stand in the kitchen as far away from the stove as possible. Take a big step forward with your right leg. Bend both knees until your left calf is parallel to the floor and your right knee is directly above (not past!) your toes. Return to standing. Switch legs and repeat, moving forward each time. When you reach the stove, if the water isn't boiling yet, turn around and go the other way.

Start Here: Recipe SuperSites

Although there are thousands of recipe Web sites online, we've picked out a few of the biggest and the best.

SOAR: The Searchable Online Archive of Recipes

```
http://soar.berkeley.edu/recipes
```

This is the mother of all recipe sites with more than 60,000 recipes in a searchable database. SOAR includes recipes for holiday cooking, special diets, camping—even recipes for your dog or cat!—as well as more than 60 regional or ethnic categories.

Meals For You

```
http://www.MealsForYou.com
```

Meals For You is undeniably one of the most useful sites on the Web for those who cook. In addition to thousands of recipes, the site offers meal plans, automatic recipe adjustments if you want to change the number of servings, and nutritional information for each recipe. You can view the recipe listings by nutrition content, preparation time, amount of calories, amount of fat, amount of cholesterol...and these are just some of the options!

The Least You Need to Know

➤ Healthy cooking has never been easier, thanks to the Internet.

➤ You can learn more about food than you ever thought possible with a few simple searches on the Web.

➤ The Internet offers an overwhelming number of recipes and cooking tips, as well as an opportunity to swap cooking hints with others.

Part 4

How to Find and Evaluate Medical Resources Online

The biggest groundswell of popular interest in the Internet is for finding medical information. The World Wide Web has opened up resources to the public that used to be available only in medical libraries or in the journals your physician received. Now you can access medical information yourself—and we show you how.

We also steer you around the tricky curves on the Information Superhighway by showing you the landmarks of credible medical sites and introducing you to some of the best ones. We teach you how to evaluate medical information so that you don't get snookered by the scams, hard sells, and malarkey that flourish online.

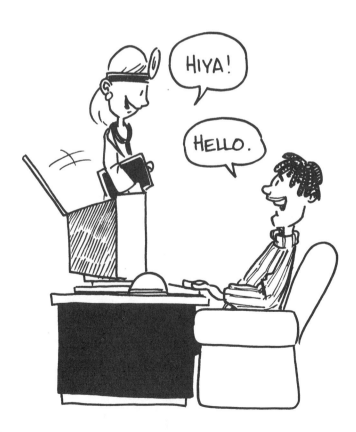

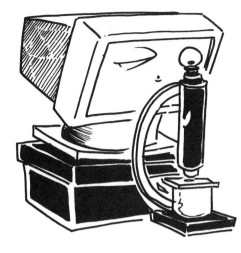

Chapter 18

Under the Microscope: Researching Health Decisions, Evaluating Medical Web Sites

---

In This Chapter

➤ Planning your search

➤ Learning how to access medical journal articles

➤ Evaluating medical information on the Web by using the PILOT method

➤ Avoiding medical quackery

There's good news and bad news about finding medical information online. The good news is that there is an almost unlimited amount of information. The bad news is that there is an almost unlimited amount of information!

You can get an unfamiliar medical diagnosis one day, and before your next appointment (or by the next day, depending on your determination and stamina), you might know more about your condition than most health professionals, including your own doctor. You can read the same research studies that your doctor does (or would, if he or she had time), search medical libraries, and "talk" to other patients with that the same condition. But be cautious—because you don't have the medical background to evaluate the information you find, you might also be swayed by unproven treatments and bilked by conwebs (we just invented that word: Web sites run by con men and con women). This chapter serves as your seeing-eye dog, guiding you through your first steps toward researching a medical topic. Then we PILOT you through your journey.

Personal Exam: What Are You Looking For?

Searching the Internet for medical information shouldn't be a passive process. There's too much of it, and if you're a passive recipient, it spills onto your screen and into your brain willy-nilly, like a huge garbage truck (actually, it's more like miles of garbage trucks) dumping its entire load onto your front lawn. Yes, treasures are buried there, but you might have to sift through piles of junk and garbage to find them, and if you're not paying attention, you might miss them altogether. You're more likely to find what you're looking for if you have a plan.

First, identify your needs and goals. You wouldn't make a doctor's appointment without knowing what you want to accomplish, whether it's evaluating a health condition, diagnosing a symptom, or curing an ache, pain, or wheeze. Likewise, although you could spend weeks just browsing one medical site after another and gathering intriguing bits of information like a wildflower bouquet, the process works better if you know what you're looking for and set your sights (and sites) in that direction.

Your best guide to medical information is your own health professional who knows your medical history firsthand. Make your own physician your ally, not your adversary, in your search for information. Start by making notes on the information your doctor has already given you, including any pamphlets or other handouts. If possible, phone your doctor and tell him or her that you're searching for information online. If your physician is computer savvy, he or she can tell you about some reliable sites to start with, and some creepy ones to avoid.

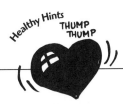

Your Question List: What Are You Hoping to Learn?

Unless you're one of those people who absolutely detests making lists, a question list can help you stay on track before you start surfing the vast Web.

For example, let's say you're a perimenopausal woman suffering from hot flashes. You set the thermostat at a comfy 55 degrees, and the family wears mittens and wool hats to dinner and begs you through chattering teeth to turn it up to 70. Your question list might look something like this:

1. What causes hot flashes?
2. How do I get cool without moving to Antarctica?
3. Will these go away if I just wait? How long?
4. Will I still have a family if I wait?
5. Do I want to get hormone replacement therapy?
6. If so, what do I need to know about the risks/benefits of estrogen? Progestin?
7. If I want to do this naturally, what are my alternatives, and how do I choose?
8. Are hot flashes influenced by diet?
9. Should I eat more soy?
10. I've heard of natural progesterone—how do I find out more about it?
11. Can I get relief with herbs?
12. How do other women decide what to do?

If these questions are uncanny replicas of your own, you'll find some sites to quench your appetite for knowledge in Chapter 23, "Menopause." Whatever your topic, when you know what you're looking for, you're more likely to find it easily.

How to Find—And Understand—Medical Journals

All Internet-based information is *not* created equal, and nowhere is that more important than in the medical field. You can find the information that physicians read to stay current, and you can find hogwash...and everything in between.

The number one source of credible medical knowledge is where doctors themselves go for information: the medical journals. Some, such as *The British Medical Journal*, http://www.bmj.com, post their articles online. Others post the table of contents and abstracts, but not the whole text of articles. Others charge a per-article fee, and it's usually well worth the small expense to learn about a study that is exactly on target.

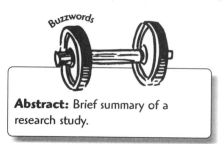

Buzzwords

Abstract: Brief summary of a research study.

Hot Links

Medline

www.nlm.nih.gov

The world's largest medical database is now free! Medline offers 9 million summaries from the world's 4,000+ top medical journals. It is one of the best ways to search for new treatment options.

Medical journals are a challenge to read and even more of a challenge to understand. They are written for health professionals, not the general public, in scientific language that is intimidating—sometimes even incomprehensible—if you're unaccustomed to reading this kind of material. Don't panic. Let the abstract and the conclusions/discussion, which are easier to understand, get you started.

These are a couple of major medical journals that offer partial online access for nonsubscribers.

Journal of the American Medical Association

http://www.jama.com

Click **This week in JAMA** for abstracts from the current issue, or click **Current Issue Table of Contents**. You can also look up past issues by date. JAMA also includes a Patient Page in each issue that you can read in full.

The New England Journal of Medicine

http://www.nejm.org

Read abstracts, tables of contents, correspondence, editorials, and book reviews for free each week. You can buy full-text individual articles, or, if you're a subscriber, you can read it all online (see Figure 18.1).

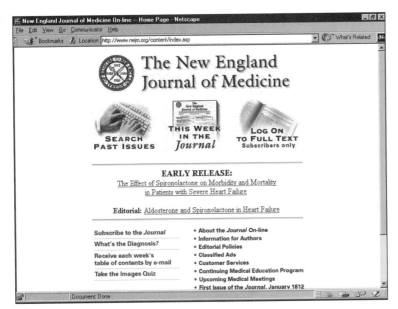

Figure 18.1

The New England Journal of Medicine Web site enables you to search past issues.

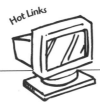

Hot Links

Your Own Medical Librarian

If you want a quick course in how to find and read medical journals or use Medline, and you wish you had your own medical librarian, you do. Her name is Rochelle Perrine Schmalz, MSL (Masters Library Science), and she works for you at Dean Edell's HealthCentral. You can find a list of her columns at `http://www.healthcentral.com`. Click **columnists**, then on the title of Ms. Schmalz's latest article, and from there, scroll down to the complete list of all her articles.

Medical Libraries

One of the greatest gifts of the Internet is immediate access to the best medical libraries, even at 2 a.m. or on Christmas day, and often this service is free. The following are some of our favorites.

The U.S. National Library of Medicine

http://www.nlm.nih.gov

The world's largest biomedical library in Bethesda, Maryland has more than 9 million references from medical journals all over the world. Online medical information online includes a consumer section called MedlinePlus: resources to help you research your health questions, including dictionaries, databases, the Medline journal abstract search, and much more. You can also explore today's hot topics, the latest technology, even 60,000 images (portraits, pictures of institutions, caricatures, genre scenes, and graphic art in a variety of media), illustrating the social and historical aspects of medicine.

MD Consult

http://www.mdconsult.com

Designed for medical professionals, this is a virtual library of medical textbooks and journals. You can search more than 35 leading medical books simultaneously, find full-text journal articles from 45 journals online, read about the latest developments in medicine, search for drugs, and read your choice of 2,600 patient handouts. **What Patients Are Reading** gives medical information about topics in the media, including synopses of *ER* episodes!

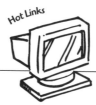

Hot Links

"How to Understand and Interpret Food and Health-Related Scientific Studies" http://ificinfo.health.org/brochure/ificrevu.htm

If you're ready to tackle the challenge of how to be an educated reader of the research, this reader-friendly article from the International Food Information Council will introduce you gently, define all the terms you need, and even tell you how to question the experts.

Buy Me: Products for Sale

We've dealt with commercial sites in detail in several other chapters, so we'll just give you a reminder here: If a site is selling products, be aware of bias in the type and slant of information you get. The information might still be valid, even excellent—a site might need to sell advertising to survive if it's not supported by other funding.

But sniff hard for any signs that the information is slanted toward product promotion, and adjust your trust meter accordingly.

The extreme "Buy Me" sites are the snake-oil schemes (not that they make it easy by labeling them as such). If a so-called medical article promotes one weird product, or is using high-powered sales tactics to get you to buy NOW!!!!, cross this site off your list. Hide your credit card, ESPECIALLY IF IT USES CAPITAL LETTERS AND EXCLAMATION POINTS!!!!!!!!

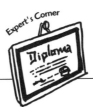

"Sites touting unproven remedies for very serious diseases, cancer, heart disease, HIV and AIDS, and particularly arthritis, are absolutely exploding on the Web."

—Jodie Bernstein, director of the FTC's bureau of consumer protection

PILOT Through the Internet

Use the PILOT Method that you learned in Chapter 3, "Junk or Jewel: Evaluating Web Site Content and Protecting Yourself," to evaluate medical sites. We'll walk you through it again, this time targeting it to medical sites.

Purpose: Why Are They Offering You This?

You're looking for sites that have one major purpose: to educate the public. Ideally, the purpose or mission is clearly stated. If not, it should be easy to interpret from the type of information presented.

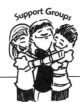

HealthBoards.com

http://www.healthboards.com

Connecting with others who have similar medical concerns can help you relate, learn, and cope. HealthBoards.com offers over 800 bulletin boards covering specific health topics where you ask questions and discuss medical issues.

Information: Content Considerations

Most consumers don't have the background to evaluate the scientific validity of medical information, but there's still a lot you can do to increase the chances that the information you're reading is helpful and accurate. Here are some questions you should ponder:

➤ How does this finding fit with other existing research?

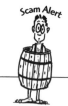

Scam Alert

Trash That Email!

Never buy a product you learn about from an unsolicited email. No cancer discovery or impotence cure will ever be announced first in a mass emailing. Scam, scam, scam.

➤ Is there a bias in this report? Are they selling the products they're endorsing?

➤ Is this fact or opinion? If it's opinion, who or what is the source, and is this opinion supported by other credible sources? Are opposing sides presented?

➤ Is this fluff or science? What research is cited? Has the research been published in a peer-reviewed journal? Are the "facts" backed by sources and references, and not simply by anecdote?

➤ Can you find the same information repeated on other sites, especially government-, hospital-, or association-sponsored sites? If the information is unique to one site, be wary!

Links: Do They Share You with Other Sites?

A site that holds you captive rather than sharing you with other sites is suspect. The best medical sites link with other sites that they've reviewed and know to be credible. But be wary of those that don't discriminate and link to anything that glows (or to those that reciprocate, regardless of quality).

Originator: Who's in Charge?

Who owns this site? Who sponsors it? Who advertises on it? Is any reputable hospital, association, or consumer agency affiliated with it? Look also at the credentials of the experts. Are they doctors or medical researchers? Are several experts quoted? Or are the so-called experts just people who have used the product and earnestly want you to benefit as they claim they have?

Timeliness: Is It Current?

Medical knowledge changes so fast that the information on a medical site *must* be current. Research is changing treatment recommendations and medications so rapidly that it's imperative to keep up. That's one of the joys of the Internet: You can see the latest data at the same time your medical professional sees it. You can read a new recommendation before it hits the newspaper. Check the dates of any article or study you read, and if the information is not based on new studies, be sure the site is updated frequently enough that if there were anything new, you'd read about it. Don't assume that just because you're at a medical training hospital site, for example, it must be up to date—a recent study found several that were not updated diligently.

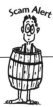

Scam Alert

Breakthrough Balderdash

Scientific breakthroughs happen in movies, not real life. Medical knowledge evolves through a long process, not sudden discoveries. Run from sites that advertise a treatment or cure that the "medical establishment" hasn't heard about yet, or "doesn't want you to know."

Ten Ways to Avoid Being Quacked

This article by Stephen Barrett, M.D., is from the QuackWatch Web site (http://www.quackwatch.com). We found it so useful that we received Dr. Barrett's permission to excerpt it here.

Promoters of quackery know how to appeal to every aspect of human vulnerability. What sells is not the quality of their products but their ability to influence their audience. Here are ten strategies to avoid being quacked:

1. Remember that quackery seldom looks outlandish. Its promoters often use scientific terms and quote (or misquote) from scientific references.

2. Ignore any practitioner who says that most diseases are caused by faulty nutrition or can be remedied by taking supplements. Although some diseases are related to diet, most are not. Where diet is a factor, the solution is not to take vitamins but to alter the diet.

3. Be wary of anecdotes and testimonials. Most single episodes of disease recover with the passage of time, and most chronic ailments have symptom-free periods. Some testimonials are complete fabrications.

4. Be wary of pseudomedical jargon. Instead of offering to treat your disease, some quacks will promise to "detoxify" your body, "balance" its chemistry, release its "nerve energy," or "bring it in harmony with nature," or to correct supposed "weaknesses" of various organs.

5. Don't fall for paranoid accusations. Unconventional practitioners often claim that the medical profession, drug companies, and the government are conspiring to suppress whatever method they espouse. No evidence to support such a theory has ever been demonstrated.

6. Forget about "secret cures." True scientists share their knowledge as part of the process of scientific development. Quacks may keep their methods secret to prevent others from demonstrating that they don't work.

7. Be wary of herbal remedies. Many herbs contain hundreds or even thousands of chemicals that have not been completely cataloged. While some may turn out to be useful, others could well prove toxic.

8. Be skeptical of any product claimed to be effective against a wide range of unrelated diseases—particularly diseases that are serious. There is no such thing as a panacea or "cure-all."

9. Ignore appeals to your vanity. One of quackery's most powerful appeals is the suggestion to "think for yourself" instead of following the collective wisdom of the scientific community.

10. Don't let desperation cloud your judgment! If you feel that your doctor isn't doing enough to help you, or if you have been told that your condition is incurable, don't stray from scientific health care in a desperate attempt to find a solution. Instead, discuss your feelings with your doctor and consider a consultation with a recognized expert.

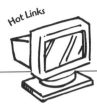

How to Evaluate Medical Information Found on the Internet

`http://new.cmanet.org/publicdoc.cfm/60/0/GENER/99`

This article from the California Medical Association combines information from the Food & Drug Administration (FDA) with additional commentary by the CMA Library staff. Most of the points are similar to our PILOT Web evaluation method, with more detail.

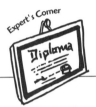

"Don't believe everything you read on the Internet. There is a difference between information and knowledge, between facts and wisdom. Ask your doctor to help you sort through what you find on the Web. Indeed, knowledge is power, but the challenge is using it wisely!"

—Holly Atkinson, M.D., Editor, HealthNews

Start Here: Super Health/Medical Meta Sites

When surfing for health and medical Web sites, stick to the most reputable. Now that you're armed with information on finding and evaluating medical and health sites, start your own research with the following meta sites and jump sites.

➤ Dean Edell's HealthCentral, `http://www.healthcentral.com/`

➤ Discovery Health, `http://www.discoveryhealth.com/`

➤ Hardin Meta Directory of Internet Health Sources, `http://www.lib.uiowa.edu/hardin/md/index.html`

➤ HealthFinder from U.S. Department of Health and Human Services, `http://www.healthfinder.org/`

➤ HealthWeb, http://www.healthweb.org/

➤ InteliHealth from Johns Hopkins, http://www.intelihealth.com

➤ Mayo Clinic, http://www.mayohealth.org/

➤ Medscape, http://www.medscape.com

➤ OnHealth, http://www.onhealth.com

➤ Mediconsult, http://www. mediconsult.com

The Least You Need to Know

➤ Medical resources vary widely in their credibility.

➤ For accuracy, read the medical journals or reliable sites that distribute and interpret their information.

➤ Use online resources in collaboration with your doctor, not instead of seeking real medical help.

➤ Remember the PILOT method to help you weed out the medical jewel sites from the junk sites.

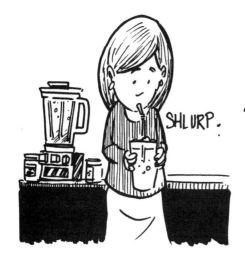

Chapter 19

Alternative Medicine

In This Chapter

➤ Finding and exploring online alternative-medicine resources

➤ Evaluating alternative-treatment claims

➤ Spotting and avoiding scams

Alternative medicine is perhaps the most controversial health area. Some people believe in it with a religious fervor. Others see the whole movement as a giant hoax. Most of us are somewhere in the middle, looking for therapies and products that hold promise and discarding those that don't. Even experts disagree about how to cleanly divide various alternative methods into "useful" and "useless," so forgive us if we wriggle out of that job, too.

Here's what we can do: We can point you to sites where you can get good information, and which seem to us to be more reliable than most. We're not endorsing or slamming any particular therapies here—we're just showing you how to explore them if you're so inclined. We can give you some potent tools for recognizing sites that are disseminating accurate information versus those just hyping their own agenda and hoping for a slice of your bank account. And we can send you to the gurus and the skeptics and let you decide for yourself.

What Can You Find?

Alternative medicine, although thousands of years old, addresses a need in our modern society. It's more personal than the 15-minute appointment and prescription we often get from our physicians. It puts us in control of our treatment and lets us participate in our healing, rather than being passive recipients. Fifty percent of patients in a recent survey said they use some form of alternative medicine. It's a blossoming field.

Alternative medicine is also known as complementary medicine, emphasizing that these different therapies can complement Western medicine and don't have to be at odds with it. Different practitioners use the handles they prefer. A new term is integrative medicine, used by health practitioners who combine alternative and Western therapies.

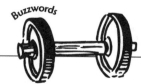

Buzzwords

Alternative/complementary medicine: A broad term covering a range of healing practices and treatments that are not generally used by physicians or hospitals, and are often not reimbursed by medical insurance companies.

The World Wide Web can quench your thirst for knowledge whether you're interested in acupuncture, chiropractic, homeopathy, hypnotherapy, reflexology, or any of dozens of other practices. The Web has opened up a world of opportunity for learning about any alternative option you could imagine and many you couldn't.

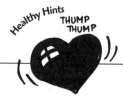

Healthy Hints THUMP THUMP

On Your Team

Before you sink money into an alternative treatment, check with your doctor, pharmacist, or other health professional. No, they are not in collusion to steer you toward expensive pharmaceuticals or medical treatments. They *are* in collusion to protect your health! You can also check out a product with the Better Business Bureau and government agencies such as your state's Attorney General, the Federal Trade Commission, the Food and Drug Administration, and, if it's sold through the mail, your Postmaster.

Just a few samples of the many alternative therapies that you can explore on the Web, with recommended "go here first" sites are presented in the following sections.

Acupuncture

Acupuncture, an ancient Chinese healing method, uses tiny needles to stimulate the nerves in skin and muscle to relieve pain and achieve other health benefits.

Alternative Medicine Therapies: Acupuncture

```
http://library.advanced.org/24206/acupuncture.html
```

What does acupuncture accomplish, how does it work, and what does it look like? Find out here, from Alternative Medicine Online, which also has pages on 20 other alternative therapies.

Ayurvedic Medicine

Ayurveda is a 4,000-year-old Indian method of healing, which believes that each person has an individual "constitution" that can be classified into three dominant types and determines a particular diet and lifestyle to achieve balance.

Ayurveda: Brief Introduction and Guide

```
http://www.ayurveda.com/info/Ayurintro.htm
```

This article from The Ayurvedic Institute by Dr. Vasant Lad is maybe the clearest explanation on the Web of what Ayurvedic medicine is, how it works, and how to apply the principles.

Chinese Medicine

Chinese medicine is a system for diagnosis, treatment, and wellness with a 23rd century track record.

Understanding Chinese Medicine from HealthWorld Online

```
http://www.healthy.net/clinic/therapy/chinmed/specifics/underst.htm
```

This information-rich site has articles on many aspects of Chinese medicine: basic principles, history, diagnosis, and how it works.

Chiropractic

Chiropractors adjust and manipulate the musculoskeletal system, especially the spinal column, to alleviate pain and imbalance.

American Chiropractic Association

    http://www.amerchiro.org/

Click **About Chiropractic** to learn what chiropractic is and read consumer tips such as how to "pull your weeds, not your back" and how to wear backpacks properly. You can also find a local chiropractor.

Feldenkrais

The Feldenkrais Method improves daily-life function by teaching the neuromuscular system new movement patterns through gentle, precise movements.

About the Feldenkrais Method

    http://www.feldenkrais.com

This site from the Feldenkrais Guild of North America not only explains the practice, but also lets you experience it with online lessons especially for computer users.

Macrobiotics

A macrobiotic diet is simple, pure, and balanced, emphasizing whole grains and vegetables and avoiding processed foods.

Macrobiotics Online

    http://www.macrobiotics.org/

This site from the Kushi Institute, a well-known macrobiotic education center, shares the philosophy of the macrobiotic way of life, disease-recovery case studies, and an assortment of recipes.

Massage

Ah, what could feel better than a massage? A good massage loosens tight muscles, releases tension, and leaves you blissfully peaceful and relaxed.

American Massage Therapy Association

    http://www.amtamassage.org/

This site explains how and why massage works, what to look for when choosing a massage therapist, and where to find one in your area (see Figure 19.1).

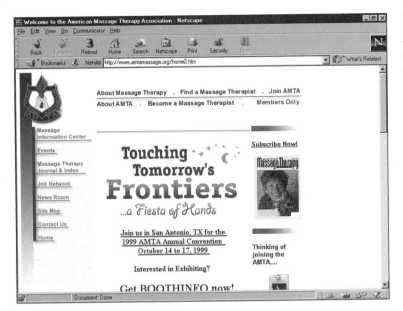

Figure 19.1

Read articles from Massage Therapy Journal at the AMTA Web site.

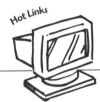

Hot Links

How to Use Alternative and Complementary Medicine

`http://my.webmd.com/topic_summary_article/DMK_ARTICLE_58289`

A helpful, unbiased article from WebMD, including research evidence, choosing a complementary therapy, choosing a practitioner, and the importance of realizing that alternative medicine is not always harmless.

Where's the Science? Fact Versus Fantasy, Opinion, and Anecdote

Many alternative therapies are popular because of opinion, anecdote, and hope. That doesn't mean they don't work, but it doesn't prove they do, either. We're not saying to wait until the research is in before getting a massage or a chiropractic adjustment when you know darn well how good these treatments feel. If your back hurts and your friend felt much better after a Reiki treatment, go ahead and try it out. We're just saying that if you're counting on an alternative treatment to treat a disease or medical condition, realize that testimonials and anecdotes aren't proof.

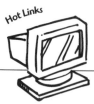

FDA Guide to Choosing Medical Treatments

http://www.fda.gov//oashi/aids/fdaguide.html

How can you tell which alternative treatment might help treat your condition, and which might make you worse (financially and physically)? This site outlines the how the FDA evaluates the safety and efficacy of a new treatment, discusses some alternative therapies that are being studied, and provides "TipOffs to RipOffs" for evaluating scam treatments.

I Believe: The Placebo Effect

One reason that testimonials are so popular in ads is that you can always find people who earnestly believe that their psoriasis cleared or their chronic fatigue lifted because of this one product or procedure. So, realize that when you hear about people who got the results you're seeking from an untested treatment, you don't know whether their improvement was actually due to the treatment, or other treatments, or spontaneous remission, or the placebo effect.

The placebo effect occurs when people take some product or undergo some process and experience a benefit because they believe they will. The mind is incredibly potent, and the power of suggestion can achieve what seem to be miraculous results. More than 30 percent of people improve with a treatment that is worthless, just because they believe in it!

"So what, as long as it works?" you might ask. But if someone else got better because of the placebo effect, you don't know whether *your* belief in the treatment will work as powerfully. Besides, if your mind is that strong, why not harness the power of your mind and heal yourself without mailing hefty checks to a placebo provider?

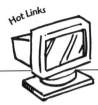

Hot Links

Separating Hype from Hope: Making Sense of Complementary Medicine Research

`http://my.webmd.com/topic_summary_article/DMK_ARTICLE_58948`

Usually there's no expert consensus on whether or not an alternative treatment works, so it's important for you, the potential user, to understand how to evaluate whatever evidence is presented. This article describes the different kinds of evidence, and how to evaluate complementary-treatment claims.

Recognizing Red Flags

The same red flags we've talked about before are waving madly in alternative-medicine scams. Hide your money and be especially wary when you see any of the following "4 C's":

➤ **Come-ons**   Words such as "secret" or "miracle."

➤ **Conspiracy allegations**   "The medical establishment/AMA/pharmaceutical companies don't want you to know!"

➤ **Cure-all claims**   There is no product or therapy that can cure everything from arthritis to zits.

➤ **CAPITAL LETTERS AND EXCLAMATION POINTS!!!!!!!!!**

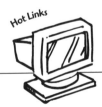

Hot Links

Bunko Squad—Quack, Quack??

`http://www.wellweb.com/altern/bunko/bunko.htm`

This bunko blaster is from the U.S. Department of Health and Human Services. It's the same information we're giving you, but maybe you're more likely to believe it if it comes from a government resource.

Start Here: Best Alternative/Complementary Sites

Many of our "Pick of the Web: Essential Health & Fitness Sites" have good alternative-medicine sections. We also recommend the following sites.

HealthWeb's Alternative/Complementary Medicine

    http://www.medsch.wisc.edu/chslib/hw/altmed/

This site from HealthWeb and the University of Wisconsin-Madison provides annotated links to numerous alternative treatments: Eastern, Western, manual, herbal, mind/body, and therapies for specific health conditions. It's all here.

Ask NOAH About: Alternative (Complementary) Medicine

    http://www.noah.cuny.edu/alternative/alternative.html

This assortment of links to a variety of alternative treatments and approaches from New York Online Access to Health (NOAH)is a good place to start exploring.

WellnessWeb: Alternative/Complementary Medicine

    http://www.wellweb.com/AlternativeComplementary_Medicine.htm

This unbiased site includes friendly advice for using complementary therapies for different conditions, with links to other sites and research press releases. Be sure to read the useful overview.

Ask Dr. Weil

    http://www.pathfinder.com/drweil/

Andrew Weil, M.D., the father of integrative medicine, answers questions and recommends natural treatments for a variety of ailments. (Although he is greatly respected in the alternative-medicine field, realize that his major sponsor is a supplement retailer, and he recommends supplements widely.)

The National Center for Complementary and Alternative Medicine (NCCAM)

    http://nccam.nih.gov

NCCAM, a branch of the National Institutes of Health, conducts and supports research and distributes information on complementary and alternative medicine (CAM). Articles on choosing and using CAM are helpful and trustworthy, although the writing style is a bit stodgy for our taste. Use the Citation Index to research specific therapies and diseases to get abstracts about research findings. (Be careful to narrow your search. A search on "asthma" and "all" CAM therapies yielded more than 2,000 reports, for example.)

Alternative Health News Online

```
http://www.altmedicine.com/
```

This is a frequently updated gateway to sites that a group of journalists consider "the most helpful alternative, complementary, and preventive health news pages on the Internet." Learn about Chinese medicine, hypnosis, naturopathic medicine, or any other familiar or unfamiliar alternative therapy (see Figure 19.2). You get news developments, warnings, consumer news, and links.

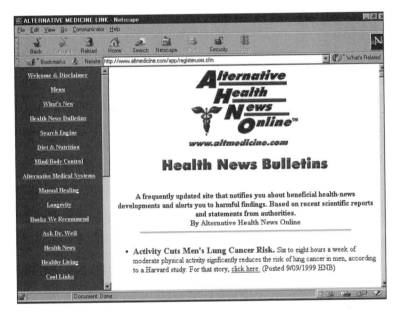

Figure 19.2

Alternative Health News Online offers news, resources, and links to plenty of alternative medicine topics.

HealthSCOUT

```
http://www.healthscout.com
```

Scroll down to **Directory** and click **Alternative Medicine** for an interesting assortment of articles—both background and news—about 17 different alternative practices, including aromatherapy, biofeedback, Chinese medicine, hypnosis, and polarity therapy.

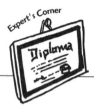

Expert's Corner

"There is no alternative medicine. There is only scientifically proven, evidence-based medicine supported by solid data or unproven medicine for which scientific evidence is lacking. Whether a therapeutic practice is 'Eastern' or 'Western,' is unconventional or mainstream, or involves mind–body techniques or molecular genetics, is largely irrelevant..."

—Phil B. Fontanarosa, M.D., and George D. Lundberg, M.D., Editorial in *Journal of the American Medical Association*, November 11, 1998

The Least You Need to Know

➤ You can locate information about any kind of alternative or complementary medical treatment on the Web.

➤ Educate yourself about what evidence supports an alternative-medicine claim.

➤ Be wary of sites that use only testimonials to promote a particular treatment.

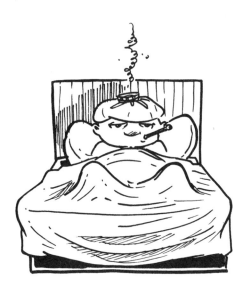

Chapter 20

Kids' Health: Illnesses and Healthy Habits

In This Chapter

➤ Finding answers online to questions about your child's health

➤ Using the Internet for advice, support, research, and education about your child's illness

➤ Using the Web to educate your children on health and fitness issues

---

Whether you are pregnant for the first time or raising your fourth teenager, you can find oodles of information online about your child's health. Many excellent Web sites that blend professional advice, research, camaraderie, and fun into useful resources for parents and kids are available for your reading pleasure. This chapter helps you PILOT through the wealth of children's health Web sites and support groups, and guides you to the best sites where you and your kids can learn and have fun.

Kids' Health for Parents

As a parent, you have questions about your child's health. What vaccinations does your child need? Is it just a cold, or is it something more serious? What can be done in the case of serious illness? And when you have healthy children—and you want them to stay that way—you want good advice on exercise, nutrition, and illness prevention.

A simple search on the keywords "parenting" or "kids' health" results in thousands of sites. These include experience-based personal pages, support, and information from other parents, magazinelike articles, and medical advice from pediatricians. As with all other health information on the Internet, use PILOT to evaluate the credibility of any site you surf.

Researching Your Child's Illness Online

When your child is ill, whether it's a minor illness or a serious disease, you want answers, options, and support. The Internet can provide all three. Of course, you still need to consult with your pediatrician, but a little research on the Web can help you fully understand your child's ailment and arm you with knowledge when choosing treatment options. The following sites are good starting points.

KidSource

http://www.kidsource.com/kidsource/pages/health.diseases.html

This site provides you with a long list of excellent articles relating to pediatric illnesses, rated to help busy parents decide which ones to read first. These cover very specific conditions, such as back-to-school with food allergies, middle-ear fluid, and teen acne.

kidsDoctor

http://www.kidsdoctor.com/

Dr. Lewis A. Coffin III used to make house calls. Now he offers advice on kidsDoctor.com, "a 24-hour-a-day source for 'What every parent needs to know'" when it comes to keeping our kids healthy." Topics include allergies, chicken pox, nosebleeds, and smelly feet (see Figure 20.1).

Figure 20.1

kidsDoctor tells you "what every parent needs to know."

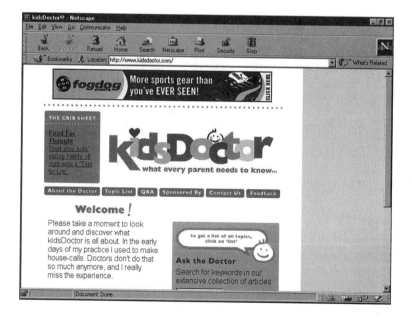

Dr. Paula

http://www.drpaula.com

As colorful as your baby's nursery, this site gives you sound information from a friendly, informed pediatrician. Rashes, sleep, sore throat, Halloween safety, head lice, diarrhea, ear wax, travel—whatever affects your child, you'll find information about it here, with dozens of articles written clearly and reassuringly. Dr. Paula Elbirt practices at Mt. Sinai Medical Center in Manhattan.

Mom's Stroller Workout

Getting a workout while caring for a small child might seem impossible, but it can be done. Put your baby in a stroller and set out for a brisk walk. At regular intervals, stop and do one of these muscle-strengthening exercises, holding onto the stroller handles:

➤ **Squats** Bend your knees, keeping your weight back as if you're about to sit in chair. Squeeze your buttocks on the way up.

➤ **Outer thigh lifts** Stand on one leg and press the other leg out to the side.

➤ **Calf raises** Rise onto your toes, and then slowly release.

Parents Helping Parents

There's nothing quite like bringing your first baby home. It's a special time, indeed, but you are no doubt nervous and unsure of yourself. When Shannon's son was born, each day presented a new challenge. She didn't want to be the mother who ran to the doctor with every little worry, but she needed some advice when she had simple questions. That's when she turned to other moms on the Internet to get answers to her questions, to commiserate when necessary, and to share her joys.

It's a wonderful feeling to know that other parents are experiencing the same things you are. Whether you are a new mom or dad, your child is suffering from a serious illness, or you are struggling to control an independent teenager, you can be sure there are other parents out there who have "been there, done that." Check out these sites for great parent-to-parent support.

ParentsPlace.com Bulletin Boards

http://www.parentsplace.com/messageboards/

ParentsPlace is a terrific site that offers hundreds of bulletin boards dealing with every aspect of parenting, including more than 75 boards devoted to kids' health issues. Topics range from asthma to vaccines.

Pregnancy Today

http://www.pregnancytoday.com (click on "the lists")

Pregnancy Today offers month-by-month mailing lists—just sign up for the month of your due date (or your child's birth if you're no longer pregnant) and join in the conversation. It's a great place to share your concerns, ask questions, and get different perspectives from others who have children the same age as yours.

Myria, the Magazine for Mothers

http://www.myria.com/lists/

Choose from more than 20 email discussion groups targeted to your child's age. You'll also find a great number of resources on mothering topics.

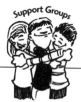

Parenting Newsgroups

In addition to the mailing lists and bulletin boards we mention, try these newsgroups for parenting support:

➤ `misc.kids.health` This active newsgroup covers all issues of kids' health.

➤ `alt.parent-teens` This newsgroup provides support for people struggling with parent-teenager relationships.

➤ `misc.kids.pregnancy` This newsgroup is a wonderful resource for pregnant and new moms.

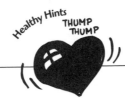

Infants Are Less Fussy When Mom Exercises

Infants whose mothers continue to exercise aerobically throughout pregnancy are more alert and less fussy than those whose moms take it easy, according to a study conducted at MetroHealth Medical Center in Cleveland. We're not sure why a mom's exercise habit affects a newborn's behavior—but it's a good reason to keep moving.

Kids' Health for Kids

Let's not grab all the online fun and education for ourselves. Give the kids the keyboard, and let them explore these kid-friendly health information sites. Young Web surfers can ask questions and learn more about their growing bodies and personal health issues at the following sites.

KidsHealth.org for Kids

```
http://kidshealth.org/kid/index.html
```

How does your body work? What makes you sick? What keeps you safe? KidsHealth.org has fun and games to help kids learn about health.

Girl Power's BodyWise

```
http://www.health.org/gpower/girlarea/bodywise/index.htm
```

Targeted to girls aged 9 to 14, this friendly and colorful site offers tips on body image, nutrition, fitness, and sports, with special sections on eating disorders, diary excerpts from female Olympic athletes, and games and puzzles (see Figure 20.2).

Band-Aides and Blackboards

```
http://funrsc.fairfield.edu/~jfleitas/contkids.html
```

With features such as "all about teasing," "hospital tour guides," and "pranks you can play in the hospital," this inspiring site helps kids deal with chronic illness and other medical problems.

Figure 20.2

Girl Power's BodyWise is "about learning to love and take care of your body."

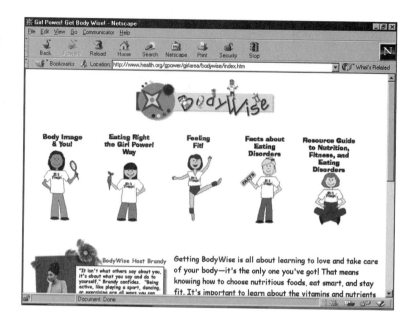

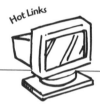

Healthy Fridge Kids' Quiz

http://www.healthyfridge.org/kids.html

Before you raid the refrigerator for some ice cream or soda, test your nutritional I.Q. with this "Healthy Fridge" quiz. As you answer each question correctly, your "fridge" fills up with nutritious foods!

Start Here: Healthy Kids' Web Sites

If you have children, these four sites should be bookmarked in your browser!

KidsHealth.org

http://kidshealth.org

KidsHealth is a magnificent site that provides in-depth information on nutrition, fitness, emotions, safety, childhood infections, immunizations, and the latest treatments (see Figure 20.3). The site is split into three sections that effectively target parents, teens, and kids.

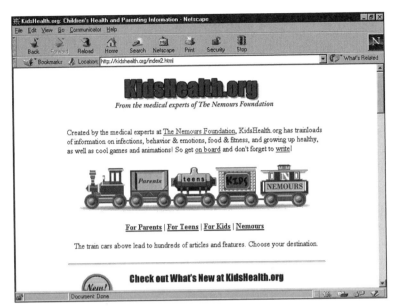

Figure 20.3

KidsHealth.org offers hundreds of articles for parents, teens, and kids. Click "All Aboard" to read them.

HealthyKids.com

http://www.healthykids.com/

HealthyKids.com is the online version of *Healthy Kids* magazine, a consumer publication of the American Academy of Pediatrics, so you're sure to find no-nonsense advice on everything from teething to temper tantrums. Choose from a bundle of message boards that put you in contact with parents who have children of the same age, single parents, parents considering adoption, or parents with special needs children.

ParentsPlace.com

http://www.parentsplace.com/health/

The Health section of ParentsPlace.com offers articles, Q & A, chats, and bulletin boards for illnesses, vaccines, development, safety, and even "adult" health concerns.

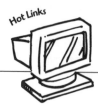

Great Expectations

For advice on everything from preconception to postpartum depression, log on the Internet and surf to these pregnancy-related sites:

Pregnancy Today

http://www.pregnancytoday.com

This site overflows with valuable information for moms-to-be and new mothers. Name your baby, develop your birth plan, read real-life birth stories, buy a good book, stay healthy throughout your pregnancy, or talk to others who have similar concerns.

Childbirth.org

http://www.childbirth.org

Do you need a doula? Should you get an epidural? Can you have a VBAC? This site is an exhaustive resource for all your pregnancy and childbirth questions.

Pregnancy at About.com

http://pregnancy.about.com/

Another quality site from About.com, here you'll find a multitude of pregnancy-related links, useful articles, due-date forums, and a gallery of ultrasound photos!

StorkSite

http://www.storksite.com

Become a "storkie" by joining this community of moms offering articles, shopping, chat, and message boards.

The Least You Need to Know

➤ Using the Internet, you can learn valuable information about your children's health, from your pregnancy through their adolescence.

➤ The Internet can guide you through a child's illness and provide support from other parents.

➤ Kids can have fun surfing the Web while learning about good health and fitness habits.

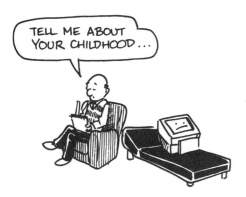

TELL ME ABOUT YOUR CHILDHOOD...

Chapter 21

Mental Health

In This Chapter

➤ Finding help in a crisis

➤ Locating information, treatment, and therapy

➤ Evaluating online therapy

➤ Getting information and support from other people who have experienced mental disorders

We all want to feel better, emotionally as well as physically. The Internet is a vast empire of information about mental health, mental disorders, and temporary but devastating setbacks such as stress and grief. If mental illness affects you, or someone you love, the Internet can't be your total solution—it's no substitute for one-on-one therapy, live support groups, or other professionally advised treatments. But in conjunction with—or preparation for—getting real, live help, it's a treasure. You can get any information you need about symptoms and treatments, and you can make friends with others who share your condition or have been through it.

Of course, the prospect of unethical money-grabbers taking advantage of your desperation is as prevalent here as anywhere on the Internet, so, please remember to let PILOT be your guide!

Mental Health/Illness Resources

If you or a loved one has been diagnosed with a mental illness or are suffering from emotional distress, you want to learn all you can, and preferably without having to whisper your problem to the local librarian. The World Wide Web is a safe haven and educational center, teaching you in the privacy of your own computer screen. You can find warm, welcoming Web sites that are helpful and nonjudgmental.

Where do you find these sites? Many of the health sites that we've applauded all the way through this book also include excellent emotional health centers with information about different mental illnesses and emotional topics, including articles, support groups, message boards, chats, and more to help you through a crisis or an ongoing problem. A good bet is to go to a few of our "Pick of the Web: Essential Health & Fitness Sites," search for the condition you want to learn more about, and start your learning there. Any of these sites can lend a friendly hand and an eye-opening journey.

In addition, this chapter points you to sites that are special jumping-off places for learning about a mental illness, its symptoms and treatments, and connections with people who have lived with similar problems. Some sites are run by professional organizations; others are run by ordinary folks who have stories to share.

Crisis Help

Your spouse dies. You lose your job. The relationship you thought would last forever ends. Your child is dangerously ill. Whatever the cause, when crisis hits with a wallop, it knocks you into an ugly, slippery black hole, and you can't find any footholds for climbing out. That's when you need crisis help. The following are some places to find it.

"Suicide: Read This First"

http://www.metanoia.org/suicide/

If you or a loved one are feeling suicidal, read this warm, earnest, and well-crafted letter acknowledging the pain and sharing strategies for getting through the crisis. This site has links to additional online resources. If you are helping a person who is suicidal, go to http://www.metanoia.org/suicide/whattodo.htm.

The Samaritans

http://www.samaritans.org.uk/

The Samaritans is a nonreligious charity founded in 1953 that exists "to provide confidential emotional support to any person who is suicidal or despairing." Trained volunteers read and reply to emails daily.

Depression

http://depression.mentalhelp.net/

"Depression is not a character flaw, nor is it simply feeling blue for a few days. Most importantly, depression is not your fault." Mental Health Net helps you understand this condition, its causes, and its treatments. The annotated links will keep you reading for days.

Death and Dying

`http://www.death-dying.com/`

Find grief support, community, and help from this site (see Figure 21.1), "designed to help you get through the hard times, meet others going through the same experiences, and find information and answers to your questions."

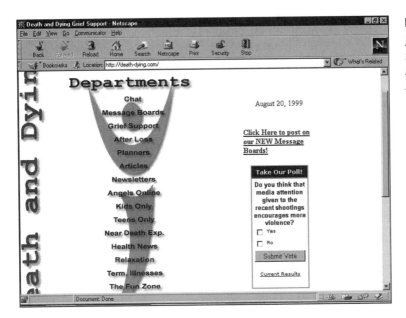

Figure 21.1

Bulletin boards, newsletters, and articles provide support and answers at the Death and Dying Web site.

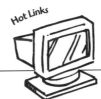

Hot Links

"Delusions About the Internet"

`http://www.sma.org/junesmj99/catalano.pdf`

This report from the Southern Medical Journal tells about people with delusions about being controlled by and entwined with the Internet, a phenomenon that the authors believe will become more common. This is an Adobe .pdf file, and you have to download the Adobe Acrobat reader if you don't already have it. If you'd prefer to read Dean Edell's reader-friendly summary, find that at
`http://www.healthcentral.com/news/newsfulltext.cfm?ID=13488.`

Exploring Treatments and Therapies

You can learn about treatments that are conventional (what a therapist or psychiatrist learns in graduate school), unconventional (alternative therapies), and downright weird. As with all types of health sites, start with the professional and consumer-advocate organizations to do your learning, and then branch out to specialized sites after you have enough knowledge to evaluate their worth. And for heaven's sake, be suspicious of any site that wants your money, unless you have reason to trust that the service is from a skilled and trustworthy professional. Put on your PILOT glasses and be wary of scam artists. For example, would you trust a site that advertises a "unique method of hypno-phone counseling that reveals your past lives from the comfort of your living room"? (That's a real site, and no, we're not sending you there.) Instead, start with the authoritative sites in this chapter, and branch out with their recommended links before exploring anything bizarre.

If you decide that therapy would be a wise idea, the Web can help you decide what you're looking for and find a therapist in your area. The American Psychological Association (http://helping.apa.org/) has a "Help Center" with information about choosing a therapist and a number to phone for a referral.

The Virtual Couch: Online Therapists

Confession time: When we first learned about cybertherapists, we said, "Yikes! Scam alert!" and figured that we would earnestly warn you to stay away from them and be done with the subject. After all, doesn't a therapist need to be able to interact with you, read your body language, coax you out of your reluctance, and notice when a facial expression indicates the need for deeper probing?

But the more we researched this intriguing issue, the more we realized that there are skilled, ethical therapists working with clients online, and there is a place for this. It's a brave new world!

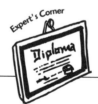

Expert's Corner

"Online therapy is very much like an interactive, self-help book. I sometimes think of it as "therapy lite." In virtual therapy, users are independent and self-responsible; they have control over when and where they engage in therapy, what they let their therapist know, and whether they will use any of the advice they get. There are many folks who have problems they could use some help with but who will not go to therapy. They might feel okay, however, about writing about their problems to a computer and getting some email advice."

—Richard Sansbury, Ph.D., licensed psychologist offering email-exchange therapy, http://www.headworks.com

Let's say you're seeking support and understanding from a trained professional, but for now, you cannot go to a therapist's office. Maybe you've never tried it before and you're too nervous or embarrassed, or maybe you live in an area where the type of therapist you need is not available. Maybe you just need to talk out your problem and get immediate advice from a trained person without committing yourself to ongoing therapy. Or maybe you need to talk to someone to find out whether your problem is serious enough to seek out face-to-face counseling.

Some issues are naturals for online therapy. Perhaps you want to write out your misgivings about a relationship, get feedback and questions, and figure out whether you want to stay or go. Or maybe you need some strategies for coping with stress. No embarrassment, no traveling to appointments, and you can write to your therapist in the dead of night when you can't sleep, or the minute after a fight with your spouse. Realize, though, that your online therapist cannot, will not, and should not diagnose or treat a mental disorder.

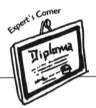

Expert's Corner

"A participant in online therapy will gain from writing—from slowing down and figuring out what is happening, sifting through his thoughts and feelings as he writes. A therapist who is reading can offer questions, insights, and options from a new perspective. Then the participant is writing again and healing himself."

—Leya Aum, M.A., Licensed Marriage and Family Therapist offering online mental health services, `http://www.sonic.net/~aumleya`

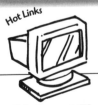

Hot Links

"ABC's of Internet Therapy"

`http://www.metanoia.org/imhs/`

Consult this guide before you decide about online therapy. It addresses how to decide whether online counseling is for you, how to protect yourself from unqualified frauds, how to evaluate therapists, and more.

Anyone can hang out an e-shingle and call him- or herself an online therapist. You can check out therapists by asking about their credentials, and then verifying these with the institutions or associations given. A shortcut is to consult Metanoia (`http://www.metanoia.org/imhs/directry.htm`), which lists online therapists and counselors and tells the types of service, credentials, methods of working, and fees of each. This site also has a list of online therapists whose credentials are in question.

If you consult an online therapist and he or she says that your problem cannot be resolved through email and advises you to get real-life therapy, please take that advice. Don't go off in a snit to the next online therapist on your list. Many problems cannot be treated online.

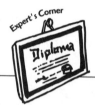

"Use care in any private online interaction with anyone. Some persons who offer email consultation or advice do not reveal their identity or their qualifications. Many of them will do so if you ask them. No online interaction is a substitute for a face-to-face interaction, and it is not currently possible to diagnose and treat disorders online. This does not mean that these interactions won't be helpful, just that they have limitations. It is important to keep these limitations in mind."

—Leonard Holmes, Ph.D., clinical psychologist, founder of NetPsychology.com (`http://netpsych.com`) and Mental Health Resources Guide at About.com (`http://mentalhealth.about.com`)

You've Got a Friend: Support Groups Online

One of the best parts of using the Internet to learn about mental illness and emotional issues is the availability of support online. Whatever your concern, you can find people who have been through it and are eager to help.

Realize, however that just having experience and eagerness doesn't make them medical authorities. Be careful to separate the emotional support that they can provide from the medical knowledge that you need to check out with authoritative sources.

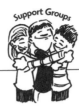

Emotional Support Groups

You'll find excellent sources of support in our "Start Here" list of the Best Mental Health Sites, but for chat, bulletin boards, mailing lists and newsgroups, try the following sites:

➤ Choose from tons of mailing lists (`http://psychcentral.com/mail-a.htm`) and newsgroups (`http://psychcentral.com/news.htm`) at Psych Central.

➤ Yahoo!'s Mental Wellness Club, `http://clubs.yahoo.com/clubs/mental-wellness`, offers chat and a message board.

➤ Chats and message boards are available at Mental Health at iVillage, `http://www.betterhealth.com/emotional/`, along with articles, resources, and experts' answers to posted questions.

Start Here: Best Mental Health Sites

Dr. Grohol's Mental Health Page

`http://psychcentral.com/`

The home page of John Grohol, Psy.D., offers mailing lists, newsgroups, links, a suicide helpline, articles, live chats, book reviews, and frequently asked questions.

National Institutes of Health

`http://www.nimh.nih.gov/publicat/index.cfm#disinfo`

If you suffer from a mental disorder or know someone who does, this section offers information about the symptoms, diagnosis, and treatment of various mental illnesses (see Figure 21.2).

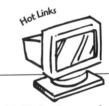

Self-Help Sourcebook

`http://mentalhelp.net/selfhelp/`

This is a guide to finding real-life (as in live people in the same room) support groups, including resources that can help you find and/or start a support group in your community.

Figure 21.2

The National Institute of Mental Health provides brochures, reports, and educational materials on mental disorders.

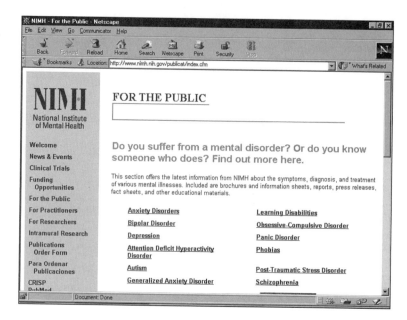

Mental Health Net

http://mentalhelp.net/dxtx.htm

Look up the disorder or problem that concerns you, and you link to both professional organizations and support groups. Even if your health problem is physical more than mental, you can get support for the emotional stress that comes with dealing with your health issue.

Mental Health Resources from About.Com

http://mentalhealth.about.com

Clinical psychologist Leonard Holmes, Ph.D., is your guide to articles, bulletin boards, and chat on a variety of mental-health issues. The annotated links make this site a good starting place—you know what to expect before you jump. Information is updated frequently.

Internet Mental Health

http://www.mentalhealth.com

"Knowledge must be shared. Our goal is to improve understanding, diagnosis, and treatment of mental illness throughout the world." A huge goal, and this site makes a good start with the 52 most common mental disorders (description, diagnosis, treatment, and research findings); the 67 most common psychiatric drugs (indications, contraindications, warnings, precautions, adverse effects, overdose, dosage, and research findings); news; magazine articles; booklets; stories of recovery; letters; and editorials. All of this from the Canadian psychiatrist, Dr. Phillip Long.

NetPsychology

```
http://netpsych.com/
```

What mental health services are available on the Internet? This site is devoted entirely to "Exploring the Online Delivery of Mental Health Services," including annotated links, news, and articles.

The Least You Need to Know

➤ You can learn about all kinds of mental disorders and emotional problems online.

➤ Although the Internet should not replace person-to-person therapy, online therapy can help you over a hurdle if you choose your professional carefully.

➤ The Web can help you choose and find a therapist and provide crisis help.

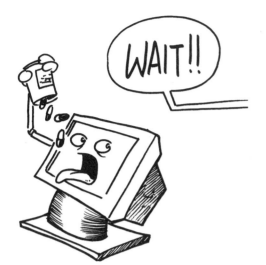

Chapter 22

Check Before Swallowing: Medication

In This Chapter

➤ Finding information about prescription drugs

➤ Exploring herbal medicine

➤ Buying drugs online

➤ Understanding the risks of self-medication and drug interactions

The World Wide Web is a powerful source of medication information. You can look up any drug—prescription, over-the-counter, or herbal—and find out everything about it, including uses, clinical studies, side effects, interactions with other drugs, and con- traindications (circumstances when this drug is not advised). Several sites even put this information into plain English! And if you want, you can order the medications you need right from the computer without changing out of your pajamas and fuzzy slippers.

This chapter shows you how to get good medication info by steering you toward rep- utable sites and bringing some caveats to your attention.

Rx: What Can You Learn?

One of the most satisfying medical uses of the World Wide Web is the ease of learning the facts about medications you're taking, considering taking, or just curious about. Whether you're comfortable reading medical lingo or need it translated into lay person's language, you can find accurate, up-to-date information. Learn what drugs are used to treat your condition and how they should be taken. Read the side effects, and check out alternatives. The more familiar you are with the facts, the more intelligently you can talk with your doctor or pharmacist. And the more information you have, the more solid your foundation is for making choices about medications.

After you've done some reading, you might need professional advice to make sense of it. A number of sites have pharmacists who answer questions online. This can be very helpful in educating yourself about the benefits and risks of certain drugs and appropriate treatments for particular medical treatments in general, sometimes including complementary treatments.

But realize that as smart and well-educated as online pharmacists and physicians might be, they don't know you, don't know what other medications you're taking, and have never examined you, asked you questions, or read your medical history. So, take the advice as general information, but consult your own health professional to ensure it applies to you.

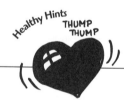

Self-Medication: Risky Business

Certainly a marvelous feeling of power and self-reliance comes from deciding on a course of action, but please do not self-medicate without consulting your personal physician or a knowledgeable pharmacist. You know your body best, but you've got to admit that your medical degree is lacking. You don't know the most current information about the drug you're considering, how it works for your medical condition, how it might interact with other drugs you're taking, and how it might affect your other medical conditions. So, don't start, stop, or cut back on a medication without consulting your physician or pharmacist. What you don't know *can* hurt you.

Buying Drugs Online

After you have a prescription for a medication, you can get it filled online. The e-pharmacy walks you through the process for getting your prescription transferred, and its pharmacist checks it. Be aware that some insurance companies do not pay for online drug purchases, so look into this before you order.

How do you know whether the online pharmacy you've chosen is reputable? Look for the VIPPS (Verified Internet Pharmacy Practice Sites) seal, being introduced by the National Association of Boards of Pharmacy to identify licensed sites in good standing. You can also be sure the seal is authentic by checking with the National Association of Boards of Pharmacy at `http://www.nabp.net`. Click **VIPPS**, and then **VIPPS list**.

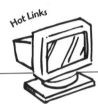

Hot Links

Confessions of an Online Drug User

`http://www.upside.com/texis/mvm/story?id=37839bc30`

Can you fill your prescriptions through the online drugstores, get your insurance to pay, and save money? Yes, no, and yes, found writer Robert McGarvey in this lively article.

Online Pharmacies

Here are some reputable e-pharmacies. Compare prices, policies, and access to a pharmacist for your questions.

➤ **CVS.com (formerly soma.com)** `http://www.CVS.com` (see Figure 22.1)

➤ **Drug Emporium** `http://www.drugemporium.com`

➤ **Drugstore.com** `http://www.drugstore.com`

➤ **Familymeds.com** `http://www.familymeds.com`

➤ **PlanetRx** `http://www.planetrx.com`

➤ **Rx.com** `http://www.Rx.com`

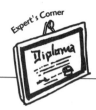

Choosing an e-Pharmacy

e-Pharmacies offer tremendous convenience and privacy, but it is critical that you know the facts about the pharmacy from which you plan to purchase products. To ensure a safe shopping experience, use these criteria when selecting an e-pharmacy:

➤ **Does the site offer 24/7 access to registered pharmacists?** Avoid Web sites that rely only on nonpharmacy personnel to answer questions, as well as those that are not willing to provide the credentials of their pharmacists.

➤ **Does the pharmacy work in cooperation with a patient's own doctor?**
Be wary of e-pharmacies or other Web sites that dispense prescription drugs based on nothing more than a "consultation" consisting of a few perfunctory questions. Legitimate online pharmacies require authorized prescriptions from a physician or authorized healthcare provider.

➤ **Is the site licensed to dispense drugs in the state where the consumer resides?** Although e-commerce laws allow legitimate companies to conduct business across state and country borders, most states have their own established guidelines and regulations. Ethical e-pharmacies are licensed in all states where they do business. To dispense Schedule II drugs (controlled substances), all e-pharmacies are required to have a federal license from the U.S. Drug Enforcement Agency.

➤ **Does the site provide reliable, objective, and up-to-date medical information?** Reputable e-pharmacies provide a wealth of free consumer information, including searchable databases of medical conditions and detailed reports on prescription drugs and their potential side effects.

➤ **Are shipping and handling costs kept to a minimum?** Carefully review the fine print to learn shipping costs.

➤ **Are safeguards in place to limit access to patients' records?** These safeguards should allow only registered pharmacists to access records and should include firewalls that alert the systems manager if a "hacker" has tried to break into the patient's database.

—Doug Callihan, R.Ph., Vice President of Merchandising and Pharmacy for the online pharmacy CVS.com (http://www.cvs.com)

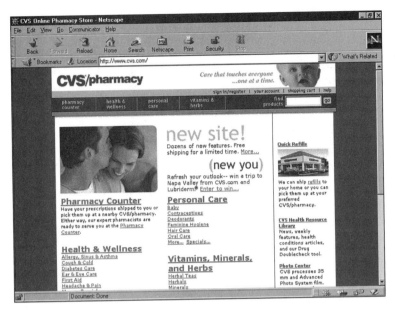

Figure 22.1

CVS.com is an online pharmacy for prescription and over-the-counter drugs, and supplements.

No Prescription, No Drug

Understand that reputable online pharmacies will fill prescriptions and provide over-the-counter drugs, but they won't provide prescription drugs when you *don't* have a prescription. This makes sense—if a medication is powerful enough to be classified prescription-only, then you should get it only after a health professional has examined you, checked your medical history, and determined that this treatment is warranted.

However, it's very easy to find disreputable or foreign sites that are willing to sell you prescription drugs without a prescription. Especially popular drugs at these sites are Viagra for sexual potency, Propecia for hair growth, Prozac for depression, and Xenical for weight loss. You have an online "examination" or "consultation" by answering a few questions, and zip, you've got a prescription. Obviously, you (or a teenager in your household) could say anything—exaggerate a condition, make up a condition—as long as the credit card number is authentic. This is dangerous—no one can evaluate whether you should get a powerful drug by collecting a few survey answers. We implore you to help stamp out these risky practices by not supporting them.

Herbal Medicine

Herbs—plants that are used for medicinal purposes—are big news. We hear their impressive benefits proclaimed by national newspapers, radio talk shows, health-food stores, and our friends. We're taking herbal supplements for a bevy of conditions, including PMS, weight loss, depression, and memory loss. There's something comforting and natural about brewing an aromatic herb tea to treat an ailment rather than popping a pill. But realize that herbs *are* medicine, and should not be used willy-nilly. Educate yourself using the Internet, but be aware—are you getting tired of hearing this?—that there's a lot of misinformation out there.

Herbal Mix Alert

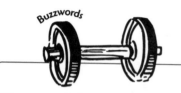

Therapeutic Interaction: The effect a drug or herb can have on a disease state; usually this is an adverse effect on a medical condition other than the one for which you are taking the medication.

Fifty percent of adult Americans are using herbal medicines, and 70 percent of those don't tell their doctor. Mixing herbs with other medications and conditions can be a recipe for disaster because of therapeutic interactions. For example, garlic can lower blood sugar, which is a caution in diabetes. Ginkgo can increase the effect of blood-thinning medications in an erratic manner. Some herbs can worsen certain medical conditions, such as saw palmetto, which can aggravate prostate cancer. Some herbs should be avoided if you are pregnant or nursing. So, talk to your doctor or pharmacist about any herbs you're considering taking.

Herbs Online

You'll find lots of herb sites on the Web—some are out to sell you and some are out to snow you, but the following sites provide substantial information. It's a good idea to check herbal information in more than one site, because few sites have everything right and up to date.

AllHerb.com

        http://www.allherb.com

Although this site is an herbal store, the information here is in-depth and invaluable. You'll find a complete reference of herbs, vitamins, minerals, and supplements (see Figure 22.2). Click **The Basics** for plain-English primers on herbs, alternative medicine, vitamins, and nutrition.

The Herb Research Foundation

        http://www.herbs.org

Scientific, political, and business news on herbal medicine. The "Online Greenpapers" highlight specific herbs and their medicinal uses.

HerbMed

http://www.amfoundation.org/herbmed.html

This research-based, comprehensive site lets you look up any herb and learn all about it, including medical uses, clinical data, toxic and adverse effects, interactions, traditional and folk use, suppliers, pictures, and plenty of scientific information. If the scientific language is daunting, take a printout to your health provider. This site does not sell products.

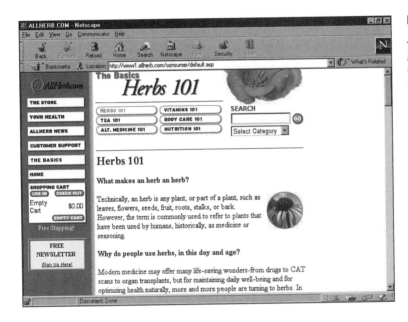

Figure 22.2

AllHerb.com offers a user-friendly site full of herbal, alternative, and nutritional information.

Healthwell.com

http://www.healthwell.com

Look up "Pharmacy" in the Health and Healing Index to read articles on herbs, supplements, herb-drug interactions, vitamins, minerals, and Western medicine. This site provides a good variety of herb articles and interesting tidbits.

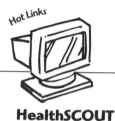

HealthSCOUT

`http://www.healthscout.com`

Scroll down to **Directory** and click **Alternative Medicine**, and then **Herbal Medicine.** You'll find about 30 interesting news articles about herbal medicine, with titles as intriguing as "Garlic Breath (why mints fail)" and "Nipping Roaches in the Bud (catnip repels cockroaches)."

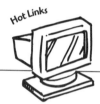

The Herbal Minefield

`http://www.quackwatch.com/01QuackeryRelatedTopics/herbs.html`

This article from Quackwatch.com tells you why you have to be careful about buying herbs to treat medical conditions: The active ingredients (with the medical properties you want) are not standardized, contents and potency are not accurately disclosed, side effects and safety might not be known or disclosed, and they might be sold by people who don't know what they're talking about.

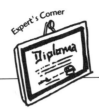

Advice from the Pharmacist

➤ **Don't buy prescription drugs online when you don't have a prescription.** These medications are prescription for a reason—they are not safe for unsupervised use! Severe side effects can ruin your life. Ask the pro football player who went into kidney failure from too much prescription-strength ibuprofen.

➤ **Tell the online pharmacist everything else you're taking.** The pharmacist needs to check for drug interactions. Along with your prescription, provide a list of all medications, OTC drugs, nutritional supplements, and herbal medications you are taking. (Take this list with you when you go to see your doctor, too!) If you use a site with no pharmacist, you are playing Russian roulette.

➤ **Ask, "Is there anything else I can do that might help?"** Do this when you're consulting a pharmacist, either online or live, about a treatment for a medical condition. Often pharmacists can recommend nontraditional treatments, such as a stress reduction class for stomach ailments.

➤ **Stick to reliable herb sites.** Otherwise, it's a crap shoot. Most sites have some good information mixed in with unreliable and often downright dangerous information. How many sites tell you not to take hawthorn products with some heart medications, for example? Do they warn about avoiding certain herbs in pregnancy/lactation? Do they list side effects? Too often, they list so many uses that you don't know the herb's common use.

➤ **Be a shrewd consumer of herbs, online and offline.** Unless you have a knowledgeable healthcare practitioner on your side, you must educate yourself about how your herbal medicines (yes, they are medicine!) will interact with your other medications and/or medical conditions. Also be wary of the product quality. One study of Asian/Korean ginseng products in North America found that 50 percent had no ginseng in them at all! Stick to the recognized brand names. They usually cost a little more, but you are worth it!

—Paul Roberts, R.Ph., clinical pharmacist at Kaiser Permanente in Santa Rosa, CA

Start Here: Drug Information Sites

You want to get the scoop on a medication and you don't want to spend your time worrying whether you're getting the right information. All these sites give accurate information in a format that's easy to find and presented in simple, lay person's language.

Personal Drugstore: Dr. Koop

```
http://www.drkoop.com/hcr/drugstore/
```

Read news about drugs, participate in chats, and check drug interactions on this authoritative site. A cool feature is the "Drug Checker" where you type in the drugs you're taking or want to know about. You can read a clear, simply worded information guide on each one, plus check interactions. Includes a directory of pharmacies that can fill your prescriptions online (see Figure 22.3).

Figure 22.3

Dr. Koop's Personal Drugstore is a one-stop site for prescription-drug information.

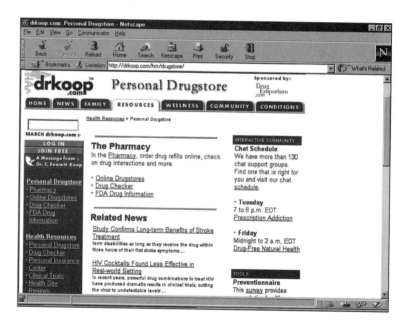

DrugDigest.org

```
http://www.drugdigest.org/
```

You can look up drugs, vitamins, and herbs; read news, research, and treatment tips; join a discussion group; and ask a pharmacist a private question. This site includes lots of information, and they're not pushing anything.

adam.com

http://www.adam.com/

If you know the medical condition but don't know what drugs to look up, this site can help. Do a search on the condition, and then click **drug leaflets** in the result type box. You end up with the same drug database used by Koop (from Multum Information Services). You might also want to read the news stories related to drugs and your disease.

Discovery Health

http://www.discoveryhealth.com

Click **Rx Central** which gives you a variety of medication pages, such as "Ask the Pharmacist," "Today's Drug News," "Recent Articles," "Disease-Specific Drugs," "Johns Hopkins Drug Commentaries," "Drug Basics," and "Poison Control." Or click **Alternative Medicine**, and then **Herbal Medicines** to learn about herbs.

iVillage allHealth

http://www.allhealth.com/

Click **drug database** to get the Medications Resource Page, where you can search by medication, browse the database alphabetically, or read articles about over-the-counter medications or the effects of certain drugs on pregnancy.

The Least You Need to Know

➤ You can find extensive information about a prescription medication online.

➤ Buying medications online can be a convenience, but check out the e-pharmacy first.

➤ Herbs are medicines and need to be carefully researched.

➤ Drugs, including herbs, can interact with one another or affect a medical condition, so get a health professional's recommendation before you medicate.

Part 5
Zeroing In: Researching Specific Medical Conditions Online

Physicians are reporting that patients are coming to their appointments carrying computer printouts on their diseases or conditions. You, too, can startle your doctor by discovering the latest treatments, reading the most current studies, and learning what experts think. We walk you through the steps to finding the best information on some of the hottest topics—menopause, HIV/AIDS, and cancer. You can then apply this process to whatever disease or condition you want to investigate.

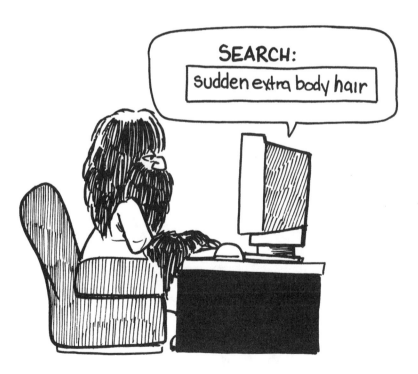

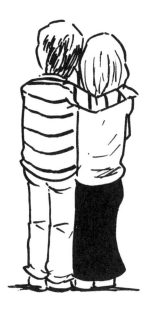

Menopause

A generation ago, women didn't talk about menopause. We're talking up a storm now. At parties, in gym locker rooms, at coffee breaks, and now online, we're discussing hot flashes, urine leaks, and vaginal dryness with as little embarrassment as we once compared diets, men, or child-rearing techniques. We're hungry for information, and we're eager to share what we're learning and our opinions about our options.

The Internet is an amazing pathway to learning the thinking of doctors, researchers, alternative practitioners, and other powersurging women, all in the same afternoon. The resources are endless, and this chapter helps you start your personal investigation and make sense of what you'll learn.

"They're Not Hot Flashes—They're Power Surges!": Symptoms

Hot flashes strike night and day. Your inner furnace blasts unpredictably while you're eating, sleeping, working, or exercising. You can be high on life one minute and in tears the next. And the...uh...er...oh, yeah, memory loss! You spend ten minutes looking for your purse (it's on your shoulder) or your keys (in the door you just opened).

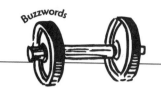

Buzzwords

Menopause: When menstruation stops permanently. A woman is said to have gone through menopause when she hasn't had a menstrual period for a year.

Symptoms might be subtle, or they might feel like PMS on steroids. They might include any assortment of hot flashes, anxiety, night sweats, insomnia, irritability, joint pains, bloating, constipation, mood swings, headaches, urinary tract problems, or a number of other imbalances. The onslaught of menopausal symptoms often appears not with the cessation of menstruation, but for a sometimes multiyear phase preceding menopause, called perimenopause.

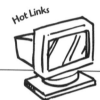

Hot Links

Self-Care Advisor: Menopause

http://my.webmd.com/self_care_article/DMK_ARTICLE_58325

This helpful article describes the symptoms of menopause, and what to do about them. Learn self-care procedures for relieving hot flashes, night sweats, vaginal dryness, and emotional stress—plus advice for when to see a doctor.

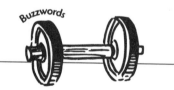

Buzzwords

Perimenopause: The years immediately preceding menopause, when symptoms have begun but menstruation has not ceased.

Treatment

To have HRT or not to have HRT, that is the question. There's a camp at one extreme that is convinced that HRT is the answer to every menopausal woman's prayers, and at the other extreme, the camp that is equally convinced that women need natural progesterone instead, or herbs and teas, or soy, or no hormone intervention at all.

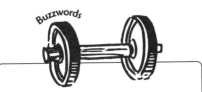

Buzzwords

HRT: Hormone replacement therapy ; the use of estrogen combined with progestin to treat menopausal symptoms and prevent some long-term effects of menopause.

Obviously, we can't resolve this issue. You're in charge of making your own decisions. Your best tactic is to educate yourself as thoroughly as possible, being rigorous with the PILOT method to identify bias and look for proof.

Even when you do this, you can't escape confusion, because there's no clear, clean, irrefutable answer to the question of which treatment is best. In another generation, we hope that the research will be more conclusive than it is now. For now, read your sources carefully and critically, and find a menopause-savvy health provider whom you can trust, because your personal health history is as important as any other factor.

Conventional

Before you decide whether you want to go the HRT route, you want to read some fair, unbiased assessments of the benefits and risks and discuss them with your health provider. One place to find this information is "Prescription Therapies" from the North American Menopause Society (http://www.menopause.org/mgprescription.htm).

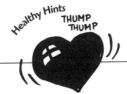

Healthy Hints

THUMP
THUMP

Menopause Doc

Ally yourself with a healthcare provider who will individualize your hormone-replacement treatment, working with you to determine the right hormones, dosages, and delivery system. You might need to try a few different drugs or alternatives, methods, and regimes.

Alternative

There's so much controversy about alternative treatments for menopause that we can't presume to sort it out for you. Which ones work? How should you take them? How do you know how much you're getting? What research has been done on these methods? You could devote the next decade to exploring these questions.

If you're considering alternatives to HRT, here are some sites that might interest you. You'll also find thoughtful alternative information in the "Start Here" and link-happy sites listed at the end of this chapter.

Menopause at Thrive

http://www.thriveonline.com/health/menopause/index.html

"Embrace the change" with Thrive, presenting "fact sheets, tools, expert advice, and lively banter." This site is friendly and spirited, with message boards encouraging you to "laugh, rant, debate, and bond," book reviews, and interviews with experts who favor natural therapies (see Figure 23.1).

Figure 23.1

Share your menopause questions and advice at Thrive.

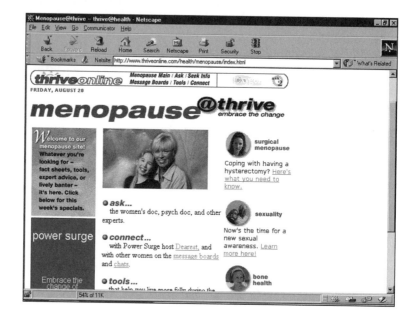

John Lee, M.D.

http://www.johnleemd.com/

Dr. Lee, the guru of natural progesterone, speaks to groups worldwide about menopause, perimenopause, PMS, and the benefits of natural progesterone over estrogen. Read his views and excerpts from his books and newsletter.

Focus on OTC "Naturals"

http://www.menopause.org/naturals.htm

This roundtable discussion published in *Menopause Management* is about what we know—and don't know—about natural progesterone creams. This was written for physicians and is not easy reading, but if you're considering these creams, you should have this information.

Support

Whom better to talk to than another sleep-deprived, irritable, hot-flashing woman, and plenty are online waiting to exchange stories and treatment suggestions.

Power Surge

`http://www.dearest.com /`

"A warm and caring community of women at midlife" created by Alice Lotto Stamm to discuss "how menopause impacts every nuance of our lives." Read guest conferences with prominent authors, and join chats and bulletin boards. Graphics-intensive site.

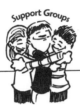

Support Groups

Menopause Support Groups

Nobody understands what a menopausal woman is experiencing like another menopausal woman. Internet support groups let you gripe, laugh, moan, and tell stories to others who are going through just what you are.

➤ Visit the Hot Flash site at `http://www.families-first.com/hotflash/`, and then subscribe to their mailing list at `http://www.onelist.com/subscribe.cgi/hotflash`.

➤ "Menopaus" mailing list:
`http://www.howdyneighbor.com/menopaus/listinfo.htm`.

➤ `alt.support.menopause` is a newsgroup for the discussion of menopause issues.

Start Here: Menopause Information Sites

The Web is full of menopause information at every general health site (look under "women's health"). Here are some special starting places where you can learn the basics and take off running.

FAQs About Menopause

> `http://www.menopause.org/faq.htm`

This site has an excellent Frequently Asked Questions section about menopause that covers not only the basics, but also detailed information about phytoestrogens (foods that contain estrogen-like properties) and different therapies.

Discovery Health

> `http://www.discoveryhealth.com`

Click **Her Health**, then **Woman and Aging**, and then **Menopause** to find a variety of articles on menopause basics, symptoms, HRT, natural therapies, and related conditions. The material is provided by Johns Hopkins, the National Institutes of Health (NIH), and other reputable sources.

Menopause Guidebook

> `http://www.menopause.org/mgintro.htm`

This online booklet from the North American Menopause Society helps you "make informed healthcare decisions at midlife." The content is extensive and conservative, pointing out where more research is needed to determine the value of particular therapies (see Figure 23.2).

Figure 23.2

Learn the basic facts about menopause from the North American Menopause Society.

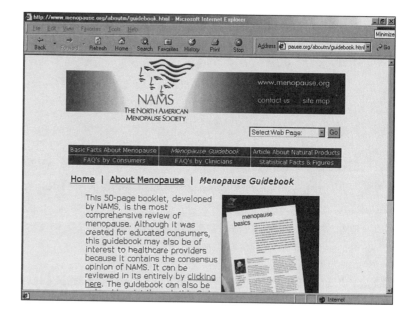

Menopause

```
http://www.nih.gov/health/chip/nia/menop/men1.htm
```

This site from National Institute of Aging explains the basics: What is menopause (the rather dry explanation spiced up with quotes from and photos of real women), what to expect, long-term effects, and hormone replacement therapy (an unbiased report of the benefits and risks, with a pro/con chart).

Doctor's Guide to Menopause Information & Resources

```
http://www.pslgroup.com/Menopause.htm
```

This site's mission is to provide "the information and information services most likely to help promote the informed and appropriate use of medicines by healthcare professionals and organizations as well as by the people to whom they are pre-scribed." You'll find "medical news and alerts" summarizing research in menopause medications, basic information about menopause and HRT, discussion groups and newsgroups, and links.

Get Linked: More Than You Ever Thought You'd Find

After you've read enough basic information to want to explore other directions, the following sites can spirit you away in any direction you care to go.

Menopause Resource Guide

```
http://www.4woman.org/owh/pub/menoguide.htm
```

The National Women's Health Information Center, from The U.S. Public Health Service's Office on Women's Health, Department of Health and Human Services, provides this guide, with many links and lists, including dozens of helpful books.

Linking Web Sites

```
http://www.menopause.org/links.htm
```

From North American Menopause Society, these links have been reviewed for accu-racy, timeliness, and consumer friendliness. None of the links are sales sites. Many are not strictly about menopause, but other related areas that you might want to explore.

The Least You Need to Know

➤ You can learn about symptoms of menopause online.

➤ The Web has many resources for exploring conventional and alternative therapies.

➤ The Internet is a gold mine of support—you share stories and questions with other midlife women.

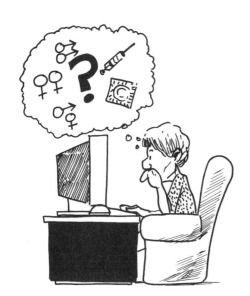

Chapter 24

HIV/AIDS

In This Chapter

➤ Learning about HIV prevention and testing

➤ Online resources for treatments and clinical trials

➤ Cautions to avoid quack cures

Maybe you don't live in one of the large cities with easy access to information about HIV/AIDS, from prevention advice and telephone hotline numbers on bus-stop posters to brochures in every library and clinic. Maybe, instead, you live in an isolated area with no easy way to get your questions answered. Or maybe you have reasons for not being able or willing to ask them. Luckily, the Internet obliterates all barriers to gathering accurate and up-to-date information about HIV/AIDS, and this chapter helps you get started.

Prevention

Prevention is the key for stopping the spread of AIDS and keeping yourself safe. You can find safer-sex guidelines, get your questions answered, and learn everything you need to "be prepared."

Prevention Tools

```
http://www.cdc.gov/nchstp/hiv_aids/prevtools.htm
```

These articles and reports from the Centers for Disease Control let you delve as deeply into prevention issues as you want. You can find the basics, read about the effectiveness of condoms, and explore a variety of related topics.

Avert

http://www.avert.org

Avert is a British educational and research charity with a mission to "prevent people from becoming infected with HIV, to improve the quality of life for those already infected, and to work with others to develop a cure." This site has a large section aimed at young people. See what you know about AIDS by taking a quiz at http://www.avert.org/hivquiz.htm.

Safersex.Org

http://www.safersex.org/safer.sex

This Web site provides readers with frank, explicit articles about the risks of various types of sexual activity, how to put on a condom, even how to talk to a partner about "smart sex" (see Figure 24.1).

Figure 24.1

Just what is safer sex? This site tells you.

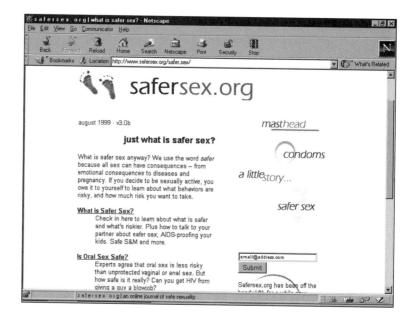

Condomania

http://www.condomania.com/safer.sex

"The Chinese made condoms out of oiled silk paper, Europeans used fish bladder, and Egyptians used papyrus soaked in water." Learn what's new in condom technology and design from this shopping site for condoms, with entertaining information you won't read anywhere else. Read condom reviews from popular magazines. Use the "Condom Wizard" to select your best brand and style. Click **safer sex**, then **educational information**, and then **manual** to read a safer-sex online booklet.

Testing

More than 200,000 Americans are unaware they are infected with HIV, according to the Centers for Disease Control and Prevention (CDC). What is the test, how do you find it, and what about anonymity? The Web gives you information about local health departments, private doctors, hospitals, and special sites that provide HIV testing. Many are anonymous—you are identified by a number. Others are confidential. Some go on your medical records and could be accessed by your medical insurance company, so check ahead of time if this is important to you. Be sure to get tested at a site that helps you interpret the test results and provides counseling.

A shortcut to finding a test in your area is the HIV/AIDS Testing site from the CDC (`http://www.hivtest.org`). This site explains and promotes early testing for those at risk. Download .pdf (readable with the Adobe Acrobat reader, available for free download online) documents about how HIV is transmitted, how to avoid getting infected, and how to get tested. Click **HIV Testing Sites** for a list of locations near you.

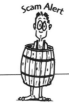

Scam Alert

Phony HIV Tests

What kind of slime would make a buck by selling phony HIV test results? The FDA recently shut down one con artist who was selling phony HIV home-test kits. Customers paid $40 and got a coin-toss diagnosis. This crook is serving five years in jail, but there are plenty more who have taken his place online.

We advise you not to go the Internet route with home-test kits, most of which give false results, according to the Federal Trade Commission (FTC). The FTC tested a variety of Internet home test kits using known HIV-infected donors. Yet every time, the kits judged the user to be healthy. As of this writing, only one home kit for HIV has been approved by the FDA: Home Access Express HIV-1 Test System. You don't get instant results with this test—you're really only *collecting* the blood at home. You mail a drop of blood on a special card to a laboratory, and then call a hotline to learn the results from a trained counselor.

Treatment

Medical advances of the last few years—particularly protease inhibitors—are extending the life expectancies of people with HIV and permitting them to live active, healthy lives. If you are HIV-positive, work closely with your personal physician to determine a course of treatment that will be best for you. Use the Internet to inform yourself so that your conversations with your physician are as useful as possible.

Do not, however, let the Internet play God. If you read about a treatment option that sounds better than anything your doctor has suggested, remember that adage, "If it sounds too good to be true, it probably is." Unless it comes from a respected medical journal or organization, take an announcement of a miracle treatment for AIDS for what it is: an ad, a come-on, a scam. Realize this: If there were a cure for AIDS, no reputable medical organization would hide it from you!

That doesn't mean that alternative treatments don't hold promise—they might. But let your doctor be your guide, and be sure to tell him or her what you're trying if you branch out on your own.

Before you try an alternative treatment, inform yourself about the medically accepted treatments at the HIV/AIDS Treatment Information Service site, http://www.hivatis.org/. The HIV/AIDS Treatment Information Service (ATIS) provides information about federally approved treatments and treatment guidelines, as well as publications and news releases, such as a warning about a home test that gives unreliable results (see Figure 24.2). A link to its sister site, the AIDS Clinical Trials Information Service (ACTIS), provides information about new treatments being studied in clinical trials.

Figure 24.2

Treatment information and guidelines are detailed at the HIV/ATIS site.

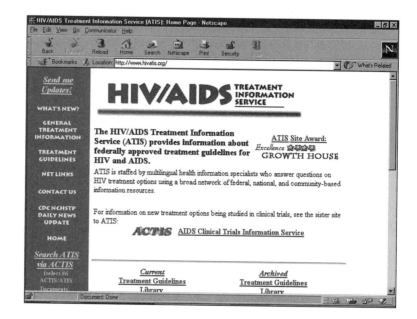

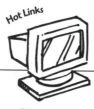

Clinical Trials

http://www.thebody.com/hivnews/aidscare/dec97/trials.html

Should you participate in clinical trials? Read the pros and cons and guidelines for deciding in an article from AIDS Care posted on The Body. Also check out "How Drugs Get Approved" (http://www.thebody.com/nmai/approval.html).

Run, Don't Walk: Spotting Quacks

Is there no end to the AIDS scams online? Treatments, nutritional supplements, mechanical devices, drugs, and even burial fees are advertised online. Fraudulent AIDS treatment products and services cost trusting consumers $10 billion annually.

Treatment scams can hurt you in several ways:

➤ The treatment, which has not been medically tested, can make your condition even worse.

➤ Even if the "treatment" is harmless, not getting the therapy you really need can do you harm.

➤ You give up your hard-earned money to these quacks.

Many quack sites advertise cures for AIDS. First, understand that no cure exists. There are treatments that can improve your health, extend your life, and improve your quality of life and comfort, but there's no cure. If there were, the medical establishment and the media would shout it from the rooftops.

A quack AIDS treatment can be recognized by these warning signs:

➤ It claims to be a "cure."

➤ The treatment is "quick," "painless," "easy," "special," "secret," "miraculous," "ancient," or "foreign."

➤ No information indicates the product's approval or side effects.

➤ The treatment is "experimental," yet you have to pay to use it.

➤ A medical establishment or government conspiracy is withholding the "truth" from you.

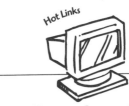

Hot Links

Ten Ways to Spot a Quack or Fraudulent Product

http://www.flairs.org/tcrs/Fraud3.htm

Use this excellent checklist from the AIDS Health Fraud Task Force (Florida) that shows you how to "investigate before you participate."

Research

If you want to know what's going on in medical research about HIV/AIDS and you're hungry for more than the news releases, but you're not ready to go straight to the medical journals, these sites can serve as your middleman.

HIV/AIDS Information Center

http://www.ama-assn.org/special/hiv/hivhome.htm

The *Journal of the American Medical Association* (JAMA) maintains this comprehensive site, including Newsline (updates, in-depth reports, and conference coverage), Library (the latest from the medical literature), Treatment Center (guidelines, treatment reviews, and resources), Education and Support Center (resources for patients and professionals), Prevention (facts, updates, and references), Policy (reviews, references, and resources), and Best of the Net (JAMA's reviewers' top site selections). Designed as a resource for physicians and other health professionals, this is not easy reading, but it's an up-to-date and authoritative resource.

The DIRT on AIDS

```
http://www.CritPath.Org/aric/dirtmain.htm
```

A quarterly online newsletter of Direct Information on Research and Treatment ("DIRT") presented by ARIC, the AIDS Research Information Center, whose mission is "Patient Empowerment Through Information." The style is academic and tight; the information is medically accurate.

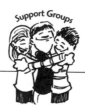

HIV Support Groups

Fighting HIV/AIDS, or caring for someone waging this war, can be easier with support. The Internet offers the comfort of "talking" to others in complete anonymity.

➤ `misc.health.aids`   This is a newsgroup for HIV/AIDS info and support.

➤ `sci.med.aids`   This is a moderated group that offers regular postings of AIDS-related magazine articles and newsletters. Postings can also be accessed through their mailing list.

➤ `http://www.thebody.com/connect.shtml`   You can find bulletin boards and chat at The Body Web site.

Start Here: HIV/AIDS Info Sites

All of our "Pick of the Web: Essential Health & Fitness Sites" have extensive information about HIV/AIDS and are excellent starting points. In addition, these sites are exceptional resources:

The Body

```
http://www.thebody.com
```

A superb AIDS and HIV resource, The Body's mission is to: "1. Use the Web to lower barriers between patients and clinicians; 2. Demystify HIV/AIDS and its treatment; 3. Improve patients' quality of life; 4. Foster community through human connection." You can read articles from the 30,000-document library, updated daily. Volunteer for clinical studies, learn about different treatments, connect to others, and get answers from experts. There's even an art gallery. This site will keep you busy for days.

HIV InSite

```
http://hivinsite.ucsf.edu/
```

This "Gateway to AIDS Knowledge" from the University of California at San Francisco AIDS Resource Institute has in-depth information about research findings, clinical trials, prevention, and social issues. Read a report about HIV/AIDS in your state or in another country. The links are diverse and plentiful. You'll find everything here.

HIV and Hepatitis.com

```
http://www.hivandhepatitis.com/
```

The aim of this site is "to improve quality of life; to slow disease progression; and to increase survival time among the hundreds of millions of people living with HIV, hepatitis B, or hepatitis C." You'll find the latest news about treatment options, vaccines, results of clinical trials, drugs, and other late-breaking reports here. You can even participate in a teleconference with medical experts who discuss treatment-related issues.

Critical Path Aids Project

```
http://www.critpath.org/
```

Founded by persons with AIDS (PWAs), this site's mission is "to provide treatment, resource, and prevention information in wide-ranging levels of detail—for researchers, service providers, treatment activists, but, first and foremost, for other PWAs who often find themselves in urgent need of information quickly and painlessly." You'll find annotated links and late-breaking news, updated daily.

HealthWeb AIDS

http://www.uic.edu/depts/lib/health/hw/aids/

This site has annotated links to dozens of selected HIV/AIDS resources. A collaboration of the Library of the Health Sciences University of Illinois at Chicago, Midwest AIDS Training and Education Center, and the HealthWeb Project.

The Least You Need to Know

➤ The Internet is a valuable source of up-to-date, credible, and confidential information about all aspects of HIV/AIDS.

➤ Use authoritative medical sites to learn about treatments and clinical trials.

➤ Be wary of the abundant AIDS scams on the Internet, especially any site that claims to have a cure for AIDS.

➤ Do not use the Internet as a substitute for medical attention from your physician.

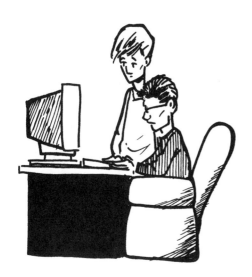

Chapter 25

Cancer

In This Chapter

➤ Finding the best online cancer resources

➤ Protecting yourself against scams

➤ Finding support online

Cancer is the most searched-for disease on the Internet. Do a search for "cancer," and you'll find 1.5 million sites. The information (and, we must say, misinformation) that abounds on the Web is so vast that we can only point you to some major resources and give you some tips for exploring on your own. After you've educated yourself and you're ready to narrow your focus, you'll find that no matter how specialized your interest, you'll find riches to mine on the Web. This chapter helps you do it.

What Can You Find?

The World Wide Web offers major sites about cancer, where you can learn about prevention, risk factors, screening, and explanations of different types of cancer. If you or a loved one has been diagnosed with cancer, you can expand your understanding of this disease, how it progresses, and your treatment options. You'll find more sites than you can visit for every type of cancer, no matter how rare, and resources on related topics. Whether you want to learn the basics of how cancer affects cells, the effectiveness of a new treatment, or alternative therapies, online resources give you virtual libraries of reading material. You can learn about and enroll in clinical trials. You can also find incredible support from Internet mailing lists, newsgroups, and chats.

Now our caveat: Beware, beware, beware. Much of the information you find is inaccurate. Recently, researchers from the University of Michigan Health System did an Internet search for information on Ewing's sarcoma, a rare form of malignant bone cancer, and analyzed a sampling of the hits. Nearly half of the 400 Web pages they reviewed contained treatment information that hadn't been medically validated (peer reviewed). About six percent gave inaccurate information, and many more were misleading. The researchers also got hundreds of dead ends, bad links, and pages with no medical information.

So, what can you do to be sure you're getting good information? Stick to the major, most reputable cancer sites (they're listed in this chapter, of course) and their reviewed links. Avoid sliding down the slippery slopes of homegrown sites for your medical information—with a few marvelous exceptions that we'll show you.

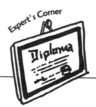

Expert's Corner

"While there are many informative sites about cancer on the Internet, there is also a good deal of unsubstantiated or outdated information online. It is tragic to see patients' survival or quality of life compromised by ill-informed decisions based on misinformation that they have gotten off of the Internet."

—Ted Gansler, M.D., director of health content for the American Cancer Society (http://www.cancer.org)

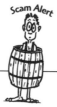

Scam Alert

Breast Cancer and Antiperspirant: The Truth

http://www2.cancer.org/zine/dsp_StoryIndex.cfm?fn=001_05211999_0

Contrary to the email that's circulating, breast cancer is not caused by antiperspirant. Read how the American Cancer Society picks apart this email line by line. The moral of the story: Never believe or circulate an email health scare without checking out the evidence at a reputable site.

Treatment Options

This is where the Internet shines. Your doctor will be impressed when you come into the office already knowledgeable about the treatments for your kind of cancer. The sites we listed as "Start Here" at the end of the chapter are your gateways to reputable information about medically approved treatments, and if your doc is Internet savvy, he or she can recommend others.

If you want to explore alternative treatments, you have to be especially careful. Yes, some hold promise, but this area is also where the scams, half-truths, unproven therapies, and repositories of wishful thinking reside. The following sites keep you on the safe side of cancer alternative treatments.

Center for Alternative Medicine Research in Cancer

    http://www.sph.uth.tmc.edu/utcam/default.htm

This site, from the Center for Alternative Medicine Research (UT-CAM) at the University of Texas/Houston Health Science Center, is dedicated to "investigating the effectiveness of complementary/alternative therapies used for cancer prevention and control." Click **Reviews of Therapies** to see research on therapies such as garlic, shark cartilage, and a macrobiotic diet. Not easy reading, but useful.

A Special Message for Cancer Patients Seeking "Alternative" Treatments

    http://www.quackwatch.com/00AboutQuackwatch/altseek.html

Quackwatch, the major watchdog site, has a special letter to cancer patients and dozens of pages about specific quack treatments. Be sure to click **Questionable Cancer Therapies**. This site is always in progress, with articles being added constantly, and Quackwatch lists the reports that aren't quite ready, as well as those that are online. Be patient if the one you want is still in progress.

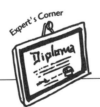

"Think at least twice before buying from any site on the Net which is engaged in the business of selling unconventional cures for serious diseases. If one of these sounds good to you, be sure to research it independently of the promoter's claims. Also, ignore all arguments about suppression of alternative therapies—this is entirely irrelevant. What is relevant is whether a therapy actually works or not, whether alternative or conventional."

—Steve Dunn, CancerGuide Webmaster (http://cancerguide.org)

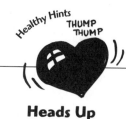

Heads Up

Be careful when viewing these types of sites, warns The American Cancer Society (`http://www.cancer.org`):

➤ Sites that are selling a product—Some sites have accurate information about chemotherapy drugs and other products that may be very useful to people with certain types of cancer. But, it is still important to ask your health care providers whether these treatments are relevant to your type and stage of cancer. Other sites promote products with no proven benefit at all.

➤ Sites provided by individual cancer survivors. Though these sites often provide valuable support and some also provide accurate and objective information, view them with caution. Some survivor's sites contain information overly influenced by their personal experience with a particular type of treatment, which may not accurately reflect whether the treatment is right for you or even for the majority of people with that type of cancer.

➤ Sites that contain information not reviewed by a medical professional.

➤ Sites that are no longer current. With all of the recent and ongoing developments in cancer, it is important to have the most up-to-date information possible.

➤ Sites that are maintained by an unfamiliar organization. Go to the most reputable organizations for accurate information.

The American Cancer Society advises you to share and validate any information gathered from the Internet with a trusted health care provider.

Support

Support groups for cancer abound, and for very good reason. People living with cancer—and the people who love them—need the compassion, information, story sharing, question exchange, and emotion venting that support groups provide.

Psychosocial Support and Personal Experiences

```
http://www.oncolink.upenn.edu/psychosocial/
```

This site from OncoLink at the University of Pennsylvania provides many support resources: books, art, and articles about sexuality, coping with cancer, coping with loss and grief, end-of-life issues, spirituality, pain management, and much more.

Share the Hope & Humor

```
http://www.cancer.med.umich.edu/share/1share.htm
```

This cancer-support site from the Comprehensive Cancer Center of the University of Michigan Health System delivers warm, compassionate writings and photography from cancer survivors (see Figure 25.1). You'll find poems, short stories, inspirational quotes and humor, and even a song.

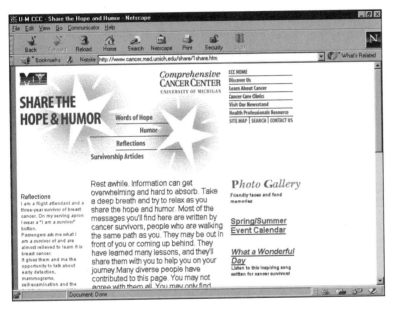

Figure 25.1

"Share the Hope & Humor" invites you to rest awhile from the overwhelming amount of cancer information found online.

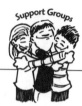

Cancer Support Groups

An average of one in four people who go online to search for information on diseases join an online support group. Here are some places to find cancer newsgroups, message boards, and mailing lists.

➤ `alt.support.cancer` This is a newsgroup for emotional and medical support.

➤ `sci.med.diseases.cancer` This newsgroup offers discussion and information on all types of cancer.

➤ `http://www.acor.org/ml/` The Association of Cancer Online Resources Inc. (ACOR) site lists more than 75 cancer information and support mailing lists.

➤ `http://www.betterhealth.com/allhealth/boards/` iVillage's Better Health site offers message boards on various types of cancers and related concerns.

How to Research the Medical Literature

We don't blame you for being intimidated by the medical literature, especially if you've never been trained to find it, read it, or understand it. Fortunately, cancer survivor and CancerGuide Webmaster Steve Dunn has invented the wheel for you in his article, "How to Research the Medical Literature" (`http://cancerguide.org/research.html`). Dunn teaches you how to use databases and online resources. This invaluable article explains different types of databases and resources, differences you'll encounter when using them, and the information you'll find from each.

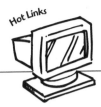

Where to Get Cancer Information Online

http://www.cancerguide.org/online.html

Starting your online exploration of cancer resources can be daunting. Your first stop should be this "tour of important Internet sites for getting basic information on your cancer." You'll learn about the three major sites, plus the best mailing lists and newsgroups.

Start Here: Cancer Info and Support

Even though we told you that you could find 1.5 million cancer sites (and that was just with one search engine), some clear winners emerge as the places to start. These sites are comprehensive and trustworthy.

American Cancer Society

http://www.cancer.org

What is cancer? Am I at risk for cancer? How can I tell whether I have cancer? What should I ask my doctor? What happens after treatment? You'll get all your questions answered at this colossal site. Read about risk factors, prevention, diagnostic techniques, the latest treatment options, alternative and complementary methods, and living with cancer, and visit ACS's bookstore.

CancerNet

http://wwwicic.nci.nih.gov/patient.htm

This is the National Cancer Institute's (NCI) Web site for cancer patients and the public. Updated monthly, all information is reviewed by oncology experts and is based on current research. The PDQ section (click **treatment information**, or go directly to http://wwwicic.nci.nih.gov/clinpdq/pif.html) lists cancers alphabetically, clearly and simply, describing prevention, detection, treatment, and supportive care for each.

CancerGuide

http://www.cancerguide.org

This site takes you by the hand and teaches you how to research your cancer. Start with "Tour of CancerGuide," which shows you how to find the specific information you want. Then explore the extensive site to learn about cancer and your situation, helpful books, confronting a difficult diagnosis, stories of other patients, clinical trials, treatments, how to research the medical literature, specific cancers, and alternative therapies. This site was created by Steve Dunn, a cancer patient from Boulder, Colorado who has done scads of work on your behalf.

Ask NOAH About: Cancer

    http://www.noah.cuny.edu/cancer/cancer.html

You'll find dozens of categories and hundreds of articles and links on this popular site from New York Online Access to Health (NOAH), providing "high-quality full-text health information for consumers that is accurate, timely, relevant, and unbiased." NOAH is a team project from the City University of New York, the Metropolitan New York Library Council, the New York Academy of Medicine, and the New York Public Library. You can read NOAH articles in English or Spanish.

OncoLink

    http://cancer.med.upenn.edu

OncoLink, a well-respected site from the University of Pennsylvania Cancer Center, has a wealth of information: specific types of cancer, medical specialties that deal with cancer, chemotherapy, bone marrow transplants, ways to cope with cancer, shared experiences of patients and survivors, causes, screening, prevention, clinical trials, financial issues, artwork, and additional resources. It's all here (see Figure 25.2).

Figure 25.2

OncoLink is a credible site with a wealth of cancer information.

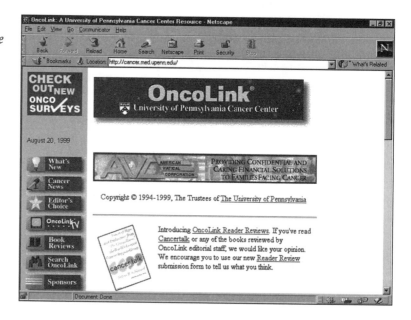

CanSearch: Online Guide to Cancer Resources

`http://www.cansearch.org/canserch/canserch.htm`

"The purpose of CanSearch is to assist online users in finding Internet cancer resources. CanSearch will take you step by step to each of the storehouses of cancer information. Many of the Internet sites are true gold mines of information." This site, from the National Coalition for Cancer Survivorship, is itself a gold mine, with reviewed resources about basic research, clinical trials, support, dealing with pain, end-of-life issues, general cancer publications, specific types of cancer, other sources of support, and gaining inspiration.

The Least You Need to Know

➤ You can find trustworthy information online about every kind of cancer.

➤ Start with the most reputable medical and cancer organizations.

➤ Be wary of treatments with unproven benefits.

➤ Take advantage of the many cancer support groups available online.

Glossary

abstract   Brief summary of a research study.

aerobic   Aerobic means in the presence of oxygen. Aerobic exercise is any activity that increases your respiratory rate and increases the capacity of the heart-lung system to deliver oxygen throughout the body. In practical terms, aerobic exercise is any rhythmic exercise using the large muscles that increases your heart rate.

alternative/complementary medicine   A broad term covering a range of healing practices and treatments that are not generally used by physicians or hospitals, and are often not reimbursed by medical insurance companies.

BMI (Body Mass Index)   A ratio between weight and height which correlates to body fat and is considered a more accurate predictor of disease risk than simply scale weight.

bookmark   When you bookmark a Web page, your computer saves the name and address of the site and keeps it in a file so that you can access it quickly at any time. Bookmarking is a great way to keep track of your favorite Web sites so that you don't have to start from scratch and search for them each time you are online or type their URL over and over.

browse   Like browsing the aisles in the grocery store, browsing the Web refers to visiting one Web site after another, looking for information that might interest you.

calories   Technically, one kilocalorie, usually called calorie, is the amount of heat necessary to raise the temperature of a liter of water one degree centigrade. Simply put, calories measure the energy produced by food in the body.

fiber   Fiber is a type of carbohydrate that is indigestible. It passes through your digestive system, helping to move other contents along. A high-fiber diet promotes a feeling of fullness, prevents various intestinal problems, and might reduce your risk of heart disease.

HRT   Hormone replacement therapy; the use of estrogen combined with progestin to treat menopausal symptoms and prevent some long-term effects of menopause.

link   Short for hyperlink; a reference to another document on the World Wide Web. Links are highlighted lines of text that take you to a Web site when you click them with your mouse.

menopause   When menstruation stops permanently. A woman is said to have gone through menopause when she hasn't had a menstrual period for a year.

metabolic rate   The rate at which you burn calories. This varies from person to person, and is raised by physical activity and by amount of muscle mass.

mind/body   Exercise technique that incorporates deep breathing, mental focus, and visualization to result in stress reduction, motivation, and enhanced physical performance.

perimenopause   The years immediately preceding menopause, when symptoms have begun but menstruation has not ceased.

placebo   A drug or other preparation that has no real medicinal effect but is given for its psychological effect on the patient.

placebo effect   The effect patients who believe a substance will work often experience when they get better although their recovery has nothing to do with what the substance contains.

quack   Medically unsound and/or promises something it doesn't deliver.

rep   A single repetition of a weight-training exercise.

resting heart rate   The number of beats per minute your heart beats at rest. The lower the number, the more efficient your heart.

resting metabolic rate   The calories you burn at rest, meaning the calories required to keep your organs working if you don't move a muscle all day. (We don't recommend that, however.)

search engine   A Web site that takes a word or phrase that you've typed and searches the Web for sites that relate to your query.

sedentary   Physically inactive, a word used to categorize (and embarrass) people who don't exercise.

set   A series of reps performed without rest.

set point   Theoretically, a mechanism that sets your weight range, similar to a thermostat. You carry a certain amount of weight that your genes determine is right for your body. When your weight goes lower than your set point, your metabolism slows down so you gain the weight back.

spam   An email, bulletin board, or newsgroup message that is posted repeatedly in inappropriate places. This might include unsolicited commercial email that tries to sell you something, or derogatory messages regarding lifestyle, political views, or religion. Also known as junk email.

strength training   Working your muscles against resistance so that they become stronger.

therapeutic interaction   The effect a drug or herb can have on a disease state; usually this is an adverse effect on a medical condition other than the one for which you are taking the medication.

Index

Symbols

24-Hour Fitness Web site, 48
1999 Harris poll, 8

A

abdominal muscles, exercising, 148
About.com Web site, 21
abstracts, 186
ACE (American Council on Exercise) Web site, 84
ACOR (Association of Cancer Online Resources Inc.) Web site, 260
ACS (American Cancer Society) Web site, 256, 261
  Web sites warning, 258
ACTIS (AIDS Clinical Trials Information Service), 250

Active Videos Web site, 108-109
ActiveLog Web site, 50
acupuncture, 197
ADA (American Dietetic Association) Web site, 129
adam.com Web site, 235
addresses, email, Joan Price, 162
adults, weight loss, statistics, 168
advice, online, 131-132
aerobics, 53
  calorie burnoff, 54
  cardiovascular
    health, 54-55
    machines, 62
  classes, 63-64
  cycling, 61
    exercise, 46
  scheduling, 56-57
  exertion levels, checking, 57, fitness, 42

  heart rates, target, calculating, 57
  inline skating, 59-60
  intensity, 57-58
  MHR (maximum heart rate), 57
  newsgroups, 56
  running, 60
  squash, 60
  stress reduction, 55-56
  swimming, 61
  tennis, 60
  videos, 63
  walking, 59
  weight loss/control, 55
Aerobics and Fitness Association of America (AFAA) Web sites, kickboxing, 63
Aerobics FAQ Web site, 54
AFAA (The Aerobics and Fitness Association of America) Web site, kickboxing, 63

AIDS. *See also* HIV/AIDs
  Clinical Trials
    Information Service
    (ACTIS), 250
  Health Fraud Task
    Force (Florida) Web
    site, 251
AikiWeb Web site, 91
AllHerb.com Web site,
  230-231
alt.support.menopause
  newsgroup, 243
AltaVista Web site, 15, 18
Alternative Health News
  Online Web site, 203
alternative medicine,
  195. *See also* medicines
  acupuncture, 197
  Ayurveda, 197
  Chinese, 197
  chiropractic, 197
  choosing, 199
  Feldenkrais
    Method, 198
  macrobiotic diets, 198
  massage, 198-199
  placebo effect, 200
  products, checking
    out, 196
  protecting yourself, 196
  scams, 201
Alternative Medicine
  Online Web site, 197
alternative treatments
  menopause, 241-243
  cancer, 257-258
alternative/complemen-
  tary medicine, 196
AMA (American Medical
  Association) Web site, 43
Amazon.com Web
  site, 108
America by Bicycle
  Web site, 115

American Bodybuilding
  Web site, 73
American Cancer Society
  (ACS) Web site, 256, 261
  Web sites warning, 258
American Chiropractic
  Association Web
  site, 198
American Council on
  Exercise (ACE) Web site,
  21, 58, 84
American Heart
  Association Web
  site, 141
American Institute for
  Cancer Research Web
  site, 21
American Massage
  Therapy Association
  (AMTA) Web site, 198
  *Message Therapy
    Journal*, 199
American Medical
  Association (AMA) Web
  site, 43
  strength training, 71
American Psychological
  Association (APA) Web
  site, 218
AMTA (American Massage
  Therapy Association)
  Web site, 198
  *Massage Therapy
    Journal*, 199
Anderson, Bob, 88
Angell, Marcia, 167
Ansfield, Alice, 170
anxiety, reducing,
  strength training, 66
Any Swing Goes Web
  site, 98

APA (American
  Psychological
  Association) Web
  site, 218
Appalachian Long
  Distance Hikers
  Association (The) Web
  site, 95
arms, triceps,
  exercising, 69
asanas (postures), 89
Ask Dr. Weil Web
  site, 202
Association of Cancer
  Online Resources Inc.
  (ACOR) Web site, 260
associations, 21
ATIS (HIV/AIDS
  Treatment Information
  Service), 250
Atkinson, Holly, 193
Aum, Leya, Web site, 219
Avert Web site, 248
Ayurvedic Institute (The)
  Web site, 197
Ayurvedic medicine, 197

B

BackWoods Grocery Web
  site, 96
BallroomDancers.com
  Web site, 99-100
Band-Aides and
  Blackboards Web
  site, 209
Barrett, Stephen, 37,
  161, 191
beans, 126
Bennett, Ruth, 101
Bennett, Steve, 101
Benny Goodsport Web
  site, 101-102

Berg, Frances M., 156, 160, 171
Bernstein, Jodie, 35, 189
Better Business Bureau, 33
Better Health Web site, 260
Bicycling Magazine Web site, 61
Bill Pearl Web site, 73
Blonz, Ed, 134
Blonz Guide to Nutrition, Food & Health Resources Web site, 134
BMI (Body Mass Index), 140
Body (The) Web site, 250, 253
Body Caliper Web site, 109
body composition fitness, 42
body fat, calipers, 109
Body Mass Index (BMI), 140
Body Positive Web site, 171-172
body types, weight loss, expectations (unrealistic), 139
body/mind, exercising, 85-86
    martial arts, 91-92
    Pilates, 90
    sports psychology, 92
    stretching, 87-88
    yoga, 88-89
bodybuilding, 73
Bodybuilding Jargon Web site, 73
BodyPump Web site, 63
bookmarks, Web pages, 19

books, diets, 158-160
Books-for-Cooks Web site, 179
breaks, standing, 9
breast cancer, false information, 256
Brick Bodies Web site, 48-49
British Medical Journal (The) Web site, 186
broths, chicken or vegetable, 176
Brown brothers (Ken and Ron) Web sites, 156, 158
browsing Web sites, 16
bulletin boards
    FitnessLink's Fitness Forum, 56
    ParentsPlace, 208
    spam, 23
    unmoderated, 24
    weight-loss support groups, 148-149
Burgard, Debby, 168, 171-172
burning calories, 46
burns fat scams, 161
business trips, exercising, 113
buttocks, exercising, 180
"Buy Me" Web sites, 188
buzzwords for diet scams, 162

C

calculating
    caloric needs, 124-125
    target heart rates, 57
calf shaper exercises, 146
California Medical Association Web site, 193

calipers, 109
Callihan, Doug, 228
Calorie Control Council Web site, 137, 143
calories, 123
    burning, 46
    burning off with aerobics, 54
    caloric needs, calculating, 124-125
    exercising, 9, 138-139
    fats, 126
    junk food, 137-138
    metabolic rate, 124, 137
    proteins, 126
    weight loss, 136-137, 143
CAM (complementary and alternative medicine), 202
CampUSA Web site, 96
cancer, 255
    alternative treatments, 257-258
    breast, false information, 256
    medical literature, researching, 260-261
    support groups, 258-260
    treatment options, 257
CancerGuide Web site, 257, 260-261
CancerNet Web site, 261
CanSearch Web site, 263
carbohydrates, 125
cardio exercise equipment, 105
cardiovascular health
    aerobics, 42, 54-55
    resting heart rate, 55
    machines, 62

CataList Web site, 23

CDC (Centers for Disease Control and Prevention), 249
Web site, 247

cellulite, scams to get rid of, 161

Center for Alternative Medicine Research (UT-CAM) Web site, 257

Center for Food Safety and Applied Nutrition Web site, 141

Center for Science in the Public Interest Web site, 38

Centers for Disease Control and Prevention (CDC), 249

certification, personal trainers, 79

chat rooms, 25
weight-loss support groups, 148

chicken broth, 176

Childbirth.org Web site, 212

children
health, 205-206
parents sharing experiences, 207-208
researching online, 206-207
Web sites, 209-212
weight loss, statistics, 169

Chinese medicine, 197

chiropractic medicine, 197

choreography, aerobics classes, 64

classes
aerobics, 63-64
dancing, 98-99

Club Med Web site, 116

clubs, exercise, 95-96

Coffin, Lewis A. III, 206

Collage Video Web site, 63, 108

commercial support groups
weight loss, 145-146
OA (Overeaters Anonymous) Web site, 146
TOPS (Take Off Pounds Sensibly) Web site, 146
Weight Watchers Web site, 145

commercial weight-loss programs, 142

complementary and alternative medicine (CAM), 202

complementary medicine. *See* alternative medicine

Complete Guide to Strength Training (The) Web site, 70

Complete Idiot's Guide to Losing Weight (The), 154, 159

Comprehensive Cancer Center Web site, 259

Condomania Web site, 248

Confessions of an Online Drug User Web site, 227

contents of Web sites, evaluating, PILOT method, 30-36

conventional treatment, menopause, 241

conwebs, 184

Cook's Thesaurus Web site, 174

cookbooks, online, 179

CookeryBooks Web site, 179

cooking
broths, chicken or vegetable, 176
ingredients, 173
freshness, 174-175
refrigerating, 174
substitutions, 174-175
meals
adding variety, 176-177
food safety, 177
shopping, 177
special interests, 178-179
microwaving method, 176
recipes
sharing, 178
Web sites, 180
steaming method, 176
stir-frying method, 176

Cool Running Web site, 60

Cory Everson's Guide to Working Out Web site, 52

Country Walkers Web site, 115

Craig, Jenny, 142

crawlers, spiders (search engines), 15

crisis help, mental health, 216-217

Critical Path Aids Project Web site, 253
CrossTrak Web site, 49
CSPI (Center for Science in the Public Interest) Web site, 133
CVS.com Web site, 227-229
Cyber Cyclery Web site, 62
CyberDiet Buddies Forum Web site, 148
CyberDiet Web site, 124, 142
CyberPump Web site, 74
cycling, 61

D

Dakota Fit Software Web site, 49
dancing, 97-99
Dearest Web site, 243
Death and Dying Web site, 217
Deering, Mary Jo, 32
DejaNews Web site, 24
delusions about Internet, Web site, 217
Depression Web site, 216
developing personal fitness programs, 45-47, 51-52
  health clubs versus home workouts, 47-48
Diet Buddy Web site, 150-151
Dietfraud Web site, 156
dieting. *See* weight loss
diets
  books, 158
    evaluating, 159-160

eating patterns, 153-154
Food Guide Pyramid, 130-131
fruits, recommended servings, 175
healthy, 129
scams
  burns fat, 161
  buzzwords, 162
  cellulite removal, 161
  junk mail, 159
  no diets or exercise, 162
  recognizing, 154-162
  testing, 163-164
vegetables, recommended servings, 175
weight
  genetic factors, 166-167
  healthy lifestyles, 167-169
  self-acceptance, 166, 169-172
  set point, 165-166
Direct Information on Research and Treatment (DIRT) Web site, 252
directories, Web, 16-17
DIRT (Direct Information on Research and Treatment) Web site, 252
Discovery Health Web site, 193, 235, 244
Doctor's Guide to Menopause Web site, 245

DogPile Web site, 18
Dr. C. Everett Koop, MD, Web site, 8
Dr. Grohol's Mental Health Page Web site, 221
Dr. McDougall Web site, 126
Dr. Paula Web site, 207
drkoop.com Web site, 8, 20
  aerobics, 63
  personal drugstore, 234
Drug Emporium Web site, 227
DrugDigest.org Web site, 234
drugs
  placebo effect, 157
  therapeutic interactions, 230
Drugstore.com Web site, 227
Dunn, Steve, 257, 260
Dyke, Larry, 78
Dyna-Bands, 107, 114

E

e-pharmacies
  criteria for choosing, 228
  pharmacists, advice from, 233
  prescription drugs, buying online, 227-228
  prescriptions, 229
VIPPS (Verified Internet Pharmacy Practice Sites) seal, 227

East Coast Swing Web site, 99
easy/effortless (buzzword), 162
Eating Disorders Awareness and Prevention, Inc. Web site, 169
eating patterns, 153-154
Edell, Dean, 11, 36, 154, 187, 193, 217
education, 9
  personal trainers, 79
email, 8
  addresses, Joan Price, 162
  health scares, 36
  pen pals, weight-loss support groups, 150
  personal trainers, 82-83
  spam, 23
  unsolicited products, 190
Epicurious Web site, 174
equipment
  calipers, 109
  cardiovascular machines, 62
  exercise
    cardio, 105
    Dyna-Bands, 107, 114
    treadmills, 106
    videos, 108
  fitness, shopping online, 103-109
    safety, 110
    scams, 111
  Fitness Products Council study, 104
  monitors, 109

ethnic recipes, Web site, 179
evaluating
  health information, 38
  PILOT method
    Web sites, 30-36
    weight loss Web sites, 141
  weight-loss books, 159-160
exaggerated claims, 29
Excite Web site, 15, 18
exercise
  aerobic, 46
  business trips, 113
  calipers, 109
  calories used, 9
  clubs, 95-96
  dancing, 97-99
  equipment
    cardio, 105
    Dyna-Bands, 107, 114
    treadmills, 106
  family fitness, 100-101
  fitness equipment, shopping online, 103-109
    safety, 110
    scams, 111
  hotels with gyms, 118-119
  monitors, 109
  mothers, effect on infants, 209
  organizations, 95-96
  outdoor activities, 93-95
  outdoors, caution, 97
  push-ups, 11
  resorts, 117-118
  scams, no diets or exercise, 162

sessions, length of, 47
spas, 117-118
standing breaks, 9
traveling
  hotels with gyms, 118-119
  resorts or spas, 117-118
  vacations, 113-116
videos, 108
exercising, 138-139. *See also* strength training
abdominal muscles
aerobics, 53
  calorie burnoff, 54
  cardiovascular health, 54-55
  cardiovascular machines, 62
  classes, 63-64
  cycling, 61
  exercise, scheduling, 56-57
  heart rates, calculating target rates, 57
  inline skating, 59-60
  intensity, 57-58
  running, 60
  squash, 60
  stress reduction, 55-56
  swimming, 61
  tennis, 60
  videos, 63
  walking, 59
  weight loss or control, 55
buttocks, 180
calf shapers, 146
calories, burning, 46

cardiovascular machines, 62
cycling, 61
exertion levels, checking, 57
Get Off Your Rocker, 139
health clubs versus home workouts, 47-48
inline skating, 59-60
MHR (maximum heart rate), 57
mind/body, 85-86
    martial arts, 91-92
    Pilates, 90
    sports psychology, 92
    stretching, 87-88
    yoga, 88-89
pushups, 79
quadriceps, 44
running, 60
squash, 60
swimming, 61
tennis, 60
thighs, 44, 180, 207
triceps, 69
walking, 59
exertion levels, checking, 57
experience, personal trainers, 80
ExRx Online Web site, 72

F

Facts About Weight Loss Products and Programs Web site, 155
families, fitness, 100-101
Familymeds.com Web site, 227
FAQs (Frequently Asked Questions), 21

fast (buzzword), 162
fat, calipers, 109
Fat City Web site, weight-loss gimmicks, how to report, 156
Fatfree: The Low Fat Vegetarian Recipe Archive Web site, 127
fats, 126-128
FDA Web site, Guide to Choosing Medical Treatments, 200
Federal Trade Commission (FTC), 249
    Operation Cure.All, 30
fees
    charged at Web sites, 31
    personal trainers, 80
Feldenkrais Guild of North America Web site, 198
Feldenkrais Method, 198
fiber, 125
Fit @ Home Web site, 105-106
Fit and Trim Support Group Web site, 147
Fit for Business Web site, 119
fitness
    activity Web site, 21
    aerobic, 42
    body composition, 42
    cardiovascular (aerobic), 42
    equipment
        calipers, 109
        exercise videos, 108
        monitors, 109
        shopping online, 103-111

for families, 100-101
    flexibility (range of motion), 42
    muscle strength, 42
Fitness Files Web site, 46
Fitness Motivation Web site, 66
Fitness Online Web site, 71
Fitness Partner Connection Jumpsite (The) Web site, 10, 58
Fitness Partner Connection Jumpsite's Activity Calorie Calculator Web site, 55
Fitness Partner Jumpsite Web site, cardiovascular machine workouts, 62
Fitness Products Council study, 104
    Web site, 105
fitness programs
    developing, 45-47, 51-52
    fitness
        determining, 41
        levels of, 42
        testing online, 42-44
    goals, setting, 44-45
    health clubs versus home workouts, 47-48
    online, advantages and disadvantages, 51
    online tools, 50-51
    progress, tracking with software, 49-51

Fitness Registry Web site, 107

Fitness Resource Web site, 51

FitnessLink, Find a Friend for Weight Loss Support Web site, 150

FitnessLink Web site, 52, 105, 111, 129, 140, 155
  certification organizations, 79
  mind/body exercising, 87
  Target Heart Rate Calculator, 57
  weight-loss books, evaluating, 159-160

flexibility (range of motion) fitness, 42

FNIC (Food and Nutrition Information Center) Web site, 128

Fogdog Web site, 106

Fontanarosa, Phil B., 204

food
  advice, online, 131-132
  beans, 126
  Blonz Guide to Nutrition, Food & Health Resources Web site, 134
  calories, 123
    metabolic rate, 124, 137
  carbohydrates, 125
  cooking, ingredients, 173-175
  CSPI (Center for Science in the Public Interest) Web site, 133
  CyberDiet Web site, 124

diets
  Food Guide Pyramid, 130-131
  healthy, 129
fats, 126-128
fiber, 125
freshness, 174-175
International Food Information Council, 188
junk, 137-138
Mayo Clinic Health Oasis Nutrition Center Web site, 132
meals
  adding variety, 176-177
  special interests, 178-179
minerals, 128
Mylifepath.com Web site, 124
phytoestrogens, 244
proteins, calories, 126
recipes, Web sites, 180
refrigerating, 174
safety, 177
scientific studies, 38
shopping, 177
substitutions, 174-175
Tufts Nutrition Navigator Web site, 132-133
Veggies Unite! Web site, 133
vitamins, 128
Food Finder Web site, 138
Food Guide Pyramid, 130-131
  A Guide to Daily Food Choices Web site, 136
  Web site, 130

Forum One Web site, 24, 148
forums. *See* bulletin boards
frauds. *See* scams
Frequently Asked Questions (FAQs), 21
fresh ingredients, 174-175
fruits, recommended servings, 175
FTC (Federal Trade Commission), 105, 249
  Operation Cure.All, 30
  Tips for Buying Exercise Equipment Web site, 104-105

G

Gansler, Ted, 256
genes, body weight
  factors, 166-167
  healthy lifestyles, 167-169
  self-acceptance, 169-172
  set point, 165-166
Georgia State University Web site, strength training, 71
Get Off Your Rocker exercise, 139
Girl Power's Body Wise Web site, 209-210
Global Health & Fitness Web site, 72
goals, personal fitness, setting, 44-45
Gold's Gym Web site, 48
Golden, Jane, 92

Goldenjane Web site, 92
GORP (The Great Outdoor Recreation Pages) Web site, 94-95
GoTo Web site, 18
Great Outdoor Recreation Pages (The) (GORP) Web site, 94-95
Grohol, John, 221
groups, aerobic classes, 64. *See also* support groups
guaranteed (buzzword), 162
gyms in hotels, 118-119

H

Hardin Meta Directory of Internet Health Sources Web site, 193
Harris poll (1999), 8
Headworks Web site, 218
health, children, 205
   parents sharing experiences, 207-208
   researching online, 206-207
   Web sites, 209-212
Health and Fitness Network Web site, 84
Health Central Web site, 11
health
   clubs versus home workouts, 47-48
   information, locating and evaluating, 38
   scares, email, 36
health/medical metasites, 193-194
HealthAtoZ Web site, 10

HealthBoards.com Web site, 189
HealthCentral Web site, 20, 36, 187, 193, 217
HealthClubs.com Web site, 48
Healthfinder Web site, 37, 193
Healthscout Web site, 28, 203, 232
HealthWeb AIDS Web site, 254
HealthWeb Web site, 194, 202
Healthwell.com Web site, 231
HealthWorld Online Web site, Chinese medicine, 197
healthy diets, 129
Healthy Fridge Web site, 210
Healthy Refrigerator Web site, 174-175
Healthy Weight Network Web site, 160, 171
HealthyKids.com Web site, 211
heart
   MHR (maximum heart rate), 57
   monitors, 109
   resting heart rate, 55
   target rates, calculating, 57
help, crisis, mental health, 216-217
Hendel, Chris, 29
Herb Research Foundation (The) Web site, 230
herbal medicines, 229
   buying online, 230-232
   herbal mix alert, 230

Herbal Minefield (The) Web site, 232
HerbMed Web site, 231
herbs, therapeutic interactions, 230
heredity, body weight factors, 166-167
   healthy lifestyles, 167-169
   self-acceptance, 166, 169, 171-172
   set point, 165-166
HIV and Hepatitis.com Web site, 253
HIV InSite Web site, 253
HIV/AIDS, 247, 253-254. *See also* AIDS
   Information Center Web site, 251
   phony test results, 249
   preventing, 247-249
   research, 251-252
   scams
      home-test kits, 249
      spotting, 251
   support groups, 252
   testing, 249
   tests, phony results, 249
   treating, 249-250
   Testing Web site, 249
   Treatment Information Service (ATIS) Web site, 250
Holmes, Leonard, 220-222
home workouts versus health clubs, 47-48
home-test kits, HIV/AIDS, 249
Honest Truth About Losing Weight and Keeping It Off (The), 159

hormone replacement therapy (HRT), 241
Hot Flash Web site, 243
HotBot Web site, 15, 18
hotels with gyms, 118-119
How to Increase the Amount of Fiber in your Diet Web site, 125
HRT (hormone replacement therapy), 241
hydrogenated fats, 127
hyperlinks, 9
    North American Menopause Society Web sites, 245
    PILOT method, 33

I

IDEA, The Health and Fitness Source Web site, 78
IMBA (International Mountain Biking Association) Web site, 95
individualization, personal trainers, 80
infants, effect of mothers' exercise, 209
information
    health, locating and evaluating, 38
    Internet
        education, 9
        quality of life, improving, 9
        reliability, 27
        research, 10-11
        scope of, 8-9

support, 11
unfiltered, 8
personal fitness, testing online, 42, 44
scams, protecting yourself, 28-30
information (PILOT method), 32
ingredients
    cooking food, 173-175
    freshness, 174-175
    refrigerating, 174
    substitutions, 174-175
inline skating, 59-60
institutions, 21
insurance, liability, personal trainers, 80
integrative medicine. *See* alternative medicine
InteliHealth Web site, 194
intensity, aerobics, 57-58
interactions, therapeutic, drugs or herbs, 230
International Food Information Council Web site, 38, 188
International Mountain Biking Association (IMBA) Web site, 95
International Sivananda Yoga Vedanta Centers Web site, 89
Internet. *See also* Web sites
    delusions about Internet Web site, 217
    information
        education, 9
        quality of life, improving, 9
        reliability, 27

research, 10-11
scope of, 8-9
support, 11
unfiltered, 8
research tools, 8
scams, protecting yourself, 28-30
WWW (World Wide Web), 8-9
Internet FAQ Consortium Web site, 21
Internet Squash Federation Web site, 60
IRC (Internet Relay Chat) Web site, 25
iVillage allHealth Web site, 235

J

JAMA (*Journal of the American Medical Association*), 186, 251
JanaTrains Web site, 57
Jazzercise Web site, 63
Jean-Paul Fitness Specialists Web site, 72
Jenny Craig Web site, 142
Joan Price Says, Yes, You CAN Get in Shape!, 159
Joan Price Web site, 45, 119
John Lee, M.D. Web site, 242
Journal of the American Medical Association (*JAMA*) Web site, 186, 251
journals, medical
    abstracts, 186
    researching, Medline, 186

Judo Web site, 92
Jujutsu Web site, 92
jump sites, 19
junk email (spam), 23
junk mail, diet
  scams, 159

K

Kalish, Susan, 100
Kassirer, Jerome P., 167
Keeling, Gloria, 86
Kick It Web site, 99
kickboxing, AFAA (The
  Aerobics and Fitness
  Association of America)
  Web site, 63
kids. *See* children
kidsDoctor Web site, 206
KidsHealth.org Web site,
  209-211
KidSource Web site, 206
Klurfeld, David, 132
Koop, Dr. C. Everett, 144
  Web site, 8
Kushi Institute, 198

L

L.L. Bean's Park Search
  Web site, 94
Lee, John, 242
liability insurance,
  personal trainers, 80
librarians, Schmalz,
  Rochelle Perrine, 187
libraries
  MD Consult, 188
  U.S. National Library
    of Medicine
    (The), 188

Life Form Web site, 50
lifestyles, healthy weight
  loss, 167-169
Lindy Hop Web site, 98
links (hyperlinks), 9
  North American
    Menopause Society
    Web sites, 245
  PILOT method, 33
lists, mailing. *See* mailing
  lists
Liszt Web site, 23-25
literature, medical, cancer
  research, 260-261
locating health
  information, 38
Long, Phillip, 222
Looksmart Web site,
  17-18
Losing Weight—An
  Ill-Fated New Year's
  Resolution Web site, 167
Low-Fat Vegetarian
  Recipe Archive Web
  site, 178
Lundberg, George D., 204
Lyons, Pat, 166

M

machines,
  cardiovascular, 62
macrobiotic diets, 198
Macrobiotics Online Web
  site, 198
magazines, 21
magic (buzzword), 162
mailing lists, 22
  Hot Flash
    Web site, 243
  Menopaus Web
    site, 243

moderated or
  unmoderated, 23
recipes, sharing, 178
weight-loss support
  groups, 147
Zoftig Zone, 171
martial arts, mind/body
  exercising, 91-92
Martial Arts Resource
  Page Web site, 91
massage, 198-199
Massage Therapy Journal,
  AMTA (American
  Massage Therapy
  Association) Web
  site, 199
Mattes, Richard, 143
matwork (Pilates), 90
maximum heart rate
  (MHR), 57
Mayo Clinic
  Health Oasis Nutrition
    Center Web site,
    128, 132
  Web site, 194
McDougall, John, Web
  site, 126
McGarvey, Robert, 227
MD Consult Web
  site, 188
meals
  adding variety, 176-177
  cooking, ingredients,
    173-175
  food, safety and
    shopping, 177
  recipes
    sharing, 178
    Web sites, 180
  special interests,
    178-179
Meals For You Web
  site, 180

meat, beans
  substituting, 126
medical information
  cancer, researching,
    260-261
  email, unsolicited
    products, 190
  researching, 184-185
    health/medical
      metasites, 193-194
    PILOT Method,
      189-191
    quacks, avoiding,
      191-193
    scientific
      breakthroughs, 191
medical journals
  abstracts, 186
  researching,
    Medline, 186
medical librarians,
  Schmalz, Rochelle
  Perrine, 187
medical libraries
  MD Consult, 188
  researching, 187-188
  U.S. National Library
    of Medicine
    (The), 188
medicines, 226. *See also*
  alternative medicine
  herbal, 229
    buying online,
      230-232
    herbal mix alert, 230
  pharmacists, advice
    from, 233
  prescription drugs
    e-pharmacies,
      227-229
  self-medication,
    warning, 226
MediConsult Web
  site, 194

Mediconsult.com
  Web site, 11
Medline, 186
Medscape Web site, 194
men, caloric needs,
  calculating, 124
Menopaus mailing list,
  Web site, 243
menopause
  alternative treatment,
    241-243
  conventional
    treatment, 241
  HRT (hormone
    replacement
    therapy), 241
  National Institute of
    Aging, 245
  North American
    Menopause
    Society, 244
  perimenopause, 240
  phytoestrogens, 244
  support groups, 243
  symptoms, 239-240
  treatment, 240-243
Menopause Guidebook
  Web site, 244
Menopause Resource
  Guide Web site, 245
menopause.org Web
  site, 242
mental health
  crisis help, 216-217
  resources, 215-216
  support groups online,
    220-221
  therapies, 218
  therapists online,
    218-220
  treatments, 218
Mental Health at iVillage
  Web site, 221

Mental Health Net
  Web site, 216, 222
Mental Health Resources
  About.Com Web
  site, 222
Mental Health Resources
  Guide at About.com
  Web site, 220
Mental Health Web
  site, 222
mental illness, resources,
  215-216
Mental Wellness Club,
  Yahoo Web site, 221
Menopause FAQs Web
  site, 244
message board (bulletin
  boards)
  FitnessLink's Fitness
    Forum, 56
  ParentsPlace, 208
  spam, 23
  unmoderated, 24
  weight-loss support
    groups, 148-149
meta sites (jump sites), 19
metabolic rate, 124, 137
Metanoia Web site, 219
metasearch Web sites,
  17-18
metasites,
  health/medical, 193-194
methods
  cooking, 176
  PILOT
    information, 32
    links, 33
    medical research,
      189-191
    originator, 34
    purpose, 31
    timeliness, 35
    Web sites,
      evaluating, 30-36

MHR (maximum heart rate), 57
microwaving method of cooking, 176
Mind Tools: Sport Psychology Web site, 92
mind/body exercising, 85-86
    martial arts, 91-92
    Pilates, 90
    sports psychology, 92
    stretching, 87-88
    yoga, 88-89
minerals, 128
moderated mailing lists, 23
money-back guarantees, 29
monitors, heart, 109
monounsaturated fats, 127
Montana Web site, 106
mothers, exercise, effects on infants, 209
Mrznet Web site, 97
Muscle & Fitness Magazine Online Web site, 74
muscles
    calf shaper exercises, 146
    quadriceps, exercising, 44
    strength
        fitness, 42
        training, 67
    thigh, exercising, 44, 180, 207
    triceps, exercising, 69
Myers, Michael D., 155
Mylifepath.com Web site, 124
Myria Web site, 208

N

National Association of Boards of Pharmacy Web site, 227
National Cancer Institute (NCI) Web site, 261
National Center for Complementary and Alternative Medicine (NCCAM) Web site, 202
National Food Safety Database Web site, 177
National Institute of Aging Web site, 245
National Institute of Mental Health, 222
National Institutes of Health (NIH) Web site, 221
National Pasta Association Web site, 177
National Women's Health Information Center Web site, 245
NCAM (National Center for Complementary and Alternative Medicine) Web site, 202
NCI (National Cancer Institute) Web site, 261
Nelson, Miriam E., 69
NetGrocer Web site, 177
NetPsychology Web site, 223
NetPsychology.com Web site, 220
Netsweat Web site, 107
New England Journal of Medicine (The) Web site, 167, 186-187

New York Online Access to Health (NOAH) Web site, 202, 262
NewRunner.com Web site, 60
news sites, 19-20
newsgroups, 8
    aerobics, 56
    alt.support. menopause, 243
    parent support, 208
    recipes, sharing, 178
    spam, 23
    unmoderated, 24
    weight-loss support groups, 147
NIH (National Institutes of Health) Web site, 221
NNF (Nutrition News Focus) Web site, 132
NOAH (New York Online Access to Health) Web site, 202, 262
NordiCaLite Web site, 163
North American Menopause Society, 244
    Web sites, 241, 245
Nourish Net Club Web site, 143
nutrition
    advice, online, 131-132
    Blonz Guide to Nutrition, Food & Health Resources Web site, 134
    calories, 123-124
    carbohydrates, 125
    CSPI (Center for Science in the Public Interest) Web site, 133

CyberDiet Web
  site, 124
diets
  Food Guide
    Pyramid, 130-131
  healthy, 129
  fats, 126-128
  fiber, 125
  Mayo Clinic Health
    Oasis Nutrition
    Center Web site, 132
  minerals, 128
  Mylifepath.com Web
    site, 124
  proteins, 126
  Tufts Nutrition
    Navigator Web site,
    132-133
  Veggies Unite! Web
    site, 133
  vitamins, 128

O

OA (Overeaters
  Anonymous)
  Web site, 146
OARS (Outdoor
  Adventure River
  Specialists) Web
  site, 116
OncoLink Web site,
  259, 262
ONElist Web site, 23
OnHealth Web site,
  20, 194
online
  advice, 131-132
  children's health,
    researching, 206-207
  cookbooks, 179
  products, checking
    out, 33

support groups
  bulletin boards,
    148-149
  chat rooms, 148
  email pen pals, 150
  mailing lists, 147
  newsgroups, 147
  weight loss, 147-150
therapists, mental
  health, 218-220
Online Stretches
  Web site, 88
Operation Cure.All
  (Federal Trade
  Commission), 30
organizations, exercise,
  95-96
originator (PILOT
  method), 34
Ornish, Dean, 159
  Web site, 126
Outdoor Adventure River
  Specialists (OARS) Web
  site, 116
outdoor exercise, 93-95
  caution, 97
Outdoor Explorer
  Web site, 94
Outward Bound Web
  site, 116
Overeaters Anonymous
  (OA) Web site, 146

P

parents
  children's health, 205
    researching online,
    206-207
  sharing experiences,
    207-208
  Web sites, 209-212
newsgroups, 208

ParentsPlace Web
  site, 208
ParentsPlace.com
  Web site, 211
pen pals, email,
  weight-loss support
  groups, 150
perimenopause, 240
Periodization of Strength
  Web site, 74
permanent
  (buzzword), 162
personal fitness programs
  developing, 46, 52
  fitness
    determining, 41
    levels of, 42
    testing online, 42-44
  goals, setting, 44-45
  health clubs versus
    home workouts,
    47-48
  online, advantages and
    disadvantages, 51
  online tools, 50-51
  progress, tracking with
    software, 49-51
personal trainers
  advantages and
    disadvantages, 78
  certification, 79
  education, 79
  experience, 80
  fees, 80
  individualization, 80
  liability insurance, 80
  personality, 81
  policies, 80
  professionalism, 80
  qualifications, 79
  via email, 82-83
personal Web sites, 22
persons with AIDS
  (PWAs), 253

pharmacies, e-pharmacies
criteria for
choosing, 228
pharmacists, advice
from, 233
prescription drugs,
buying online,
227-228
prescriptions, 229
VIPPS (Verified
Internet Pharmacy
Practice Sites)
seal, 227
pharmacists, advice
from, 233
Phys.com Web site, 88
PHYS: Snack Bandit
Web site, 95
phytoestrogens, 244
Pilates, mind/body
exercising, 90
Pilates-Studio Web
site, 90
PILOT method
information, 32
links, 33
medical research,
189-191
originator, 34
purpose, 31
timeliness, 35
Web sites, evaluating,
30-36
weight loss Web sites,
evaluating, 141
placebo effect, 157
alternative
medicine, 200
PlanetRx Web site, 227
Polar Web site, 109
Polevoy, Terry, 156
policies, personal
trainers, 80

Poliquin, Charles, 74
polyunsaturated fats, 127
postures (asanas), 89
Pregnancy at About.com
Web site, 212
Pregnancy Today Web
site, 208, 212
prescription drugs,
e-pharmacies, 227-229
preventing HIV/AIDS,
247-249
Price, Joan, 159
email address, 162
Pro Track 99 Web site, 49
products, checking out
alternative
medicine, 196
online, 33
professionalism, personal
trainers, 80
programs
maintenance,
choosing, 141
personal fitness, 45-46
developing, 51-52
health clubs versus
home workouts,
47-48
online tools, 50-51
progress, tracking
with software,
49-51
weight loss
choosing, 140-141
commercial, 142
progress with fitness
programs, tracking with
software, 49-51
proteins, beans or
calories, 126
Psych Central Web
site, 221

psychology, sports,
mind/body,
exercising, 92
Public Eye (The) Web
site, 110
Publicly Accessible
Mailing Lists Web
site, 23
purpose (PILOT
method), 31
push-ups, 11, 79
PWAs (persons with
AIDS), 253

Q

quacks, 28
identifying, 160
medical information,
avoiding, 191-193
weight-loss sites
Quackwatch Web site,
37, 105
cancer quack
treatments, 257
cellulite removal, 161
weight-loss
gimmicks, 156
Quackwatch.com Web
site, 232
quadriceps, exercising, 44
qualifications, personal
trainers, 79
quality of life
education, 9
improving, 9
research, 10-11
support, 11

R

Racewalk Web site, 59
Radiance Web site,
  168, 170
Randolfi, Ernesto A.,
  Web site, 38
RDs (registered
  dietitians), 129
recipes
  ethnic, Web site, 179
  ingredients, 173-175
  sharing, 178
  traditional, Web
    site, 179
  Web sites, 180
recreation
  clubs, exercise, 95-96
  dancing, 97-99
  family fitness, 100-101
  organizations, exercise,
    95-96
  outdoor activities
    exercise, 93-97
Recreation at About.com
  Web site, 95
refrigerating,
  ingredients, 174
registered dietitians
  (RDs), 129
reliability
  information on
    Internet, 27
  Web sites, 29
Renner, John H., 28
reps (repetition), strength
  training, 68
research, 10-11
  cancer, medical
    literature, 260-261
  children's health,
    206-207
  HIV/AIDS, 251-252

medical information,
  184-185
  health/medical
    metasites, 193-194
  PILOT Method,
    189-191
  quacks, avoiding,
    191-193
  scientific
    breakthroughs, 191
medical journals,
  abstracts or
  Medline, 186
medical libraries,
  187-188
tools on Internet, 8
weight loss, 140-141
resistance training,
  strength training, 65
  advantages of, 66
  anxiety reducer, 66
  basics, 67
  bodybuilding, 73
  muscles, 67
  results, 70
  scams, Web sites, 72
  scheduling
    exercises, 68
  sets, 68
  strength-assessment
    test, 70
  stress reducer, 66
  weights, 69
  for women, 67
resorts, exercising,
  117-118
resources, mental health
  and mental illness,
  215-216
resting heart rate, 55
Reuters Health eLine
  Web site, 20

Richard Simmons Web
  site, 118, 149
Rob Wood's Fitness
  Testing Web site, 43
Roberts, Paul, 233
robots (spiders), search
  engines, 15
Rollerblade.com Web site,
  59-60
rooms, chat, 25
  weight-loss support
    groups, 148
running, 60
Rx.com Web site, 227

S

SaferSex.org Web
  site, 248
safety
  food, 177
  shopping online, 110
Samaritans (The) Web
  site, 216
Sansbury, Richard, 218
saturated fats, 127
SavoyStyle Swing Dance
  Shop Web site, 98
SavvySearch Web site, 18
scams
  alternative
    medicine, 201
  Better Business
    Bureau, 33
  breast cancer, 256
  burns fat, 161
  diets
    burns fat, 161
    buzzwords, 162
    cellulite
      removal, 161
    junk mail, 159

no diets or
   exercise, 162
recognizing, 154-162
testing, 163-164
email
   health scares, 36
   unsolicited
      products, 190
fees, charged at Web
   sites, 31
HIV/AIDS
   spotting, 251
   home-test kits, 249
medical quacks,
   avoiding, 191-193
mental health
   treatments and
   therapies, 218
money-back
   guarantees, 29
personal trainers via
   email, 82-83
products online,
   checking out, 33
protecting yourself,
   28-30
quacks, 28
Quackwatch Web
   site, 37
shopping online, 111
strength training
   Web sites, 72
Web sites, look of, 34
scheduling
   aerobic exercises, 56-57
   strength training
   exercises, 68-69
Schmalz, Rochelle
   Perrine, 187
Schuler, Lou, 82
scientific
   breakthroughs, 191
   studies, 38

Search Engine Showdown
   Web site, 14
search engines, 14
   metasearch sites, 17-18
   spiders, 15
   Web directories, 16-17
Searchable Online
   Archive of Recipes
   (SOAR) Web sites,
   178, 180
secret (buzzword), 162
security, shopping
   online, 110
sedentary, 42
self-acceptance of
   weight, 169, 171-172
Self-Care Advisor:
   Menopause Web
   site, 240
self-medication,
   warning, 226
set point of body weight,
   165-166
sets, strength training, 68
Shape Up America Fitness
   Club Assessment
   Web site, 43
Shape Up America Web
   site, 101, 144
Share the Hope & Humor
   Web site, 259
shopping
   food, 177
   online
      calipers, 109
      exercise videos, 108
      fitness equipment,
      103-109
      monitors, 109
      safety, 110
      scams, 111
Sierra Club Web site, 96

Silverglade, Bruce, 38
Simmons, Richard,
   118, 149
sites, Web. *See* Web sites
skating, inline, 59-60
Skating.com Web site, 59
Ski Travel Online Web
   site, 116
SkiCentral Web site, 96
Snack Bandit Web site, 95
Snap Web site, 17-18
SOAR (Searchable Online
   Archive of Recipes) Web
   site, 178, 180
social dancing, 98-99
software, personal fitness
   programs, tracking
   progress, 49-51
soma.com, CVS.com Web
   site, 227-229
Something Fishy Web site
   on Eating Disorders
   (The) Web site, 169
Southern Medical Journal
   Web site, 217
Spa Magazine
   Web site, 118
Spa-Finder Web site, 117
spam, 23
spas, exercising, 117-118
spiders, search
   engines, 15
Spinning Web site, 63
Sports Parents
   Web site, 101
sports psychology,
   mind/body
   exercising, 92
squash, World Squash
   Federation, 60
Stamm, Alice Lotto, 243
standing breaks, 9

StarChefs Web site, 179
statistics, weight loss
adults, 168
children, 169
steaming method of
cooking, 176
stir-frying method of
cooking, 176
storefront Web sites, 22
StorkSite Web site, 212
Stott Conditioning Web
site, 90
STOTT Pilates Studios &
International
Certification Center
Web site, 90
Stott, Moira, 90
strength training, 65. *See
also* exercising
advantages of, 66
anxiety reducer, 66
basics, 67
bodybuilding, 73
muscles, 67
results, 70
scams, Web sites, 72
scheduling
exercises, 68
sets, 68
strength-assessment
test, 70
stress reducer, 66
weights, 69
for women, 67
Strength Training and
Women Web site, 67
strength-assessment test,
Web site, 70
stress, reducing, 55-56
strength training, 66
stretching, mind/body
exercising, 87-88
Strong Women Web
site, 69

Strong, Stretched &
Centered Mind-Body
Fitness Training
Institute Web site, 86
substitutions, ingredients,
174-175
Suicide: Read This First
Web site, 216
suitcases, lifting
properly, 119
support groups, 11
cancer, 258, 260
HIV/AIDS, 252
menopause, 243
mental health, 220-221
newsgroups, for
parents, 208
online, mental health,
220-221
weight loss
bulletin boards,
148-149
chat rooms, 148
commercial, 145-146
email pen pals, 150
mailing lists, 147
newsgroups, 147
OA (Overeaters
Anonymous) Web
site, 146
online, 147-150
TOPS (Take Off
Pounds Sensibly)
Web site, 146
Weight Watchers
Web site, 145
Swan, Jay, 91
Swim 2000 Web site, 61
SwimInfo Web site, 61
swimming, 61
Switcheroo Web site, 174
symptoms, menopause,
239-240

T

Tai Chi Web site, 92
Tanita Web site, 109
target heart rates,
calculating, 57
tennis, 60
TennisLinks.com
Web site, 60
testing
diet scams, 163-164
HIV/AIDS, 249
personal fitness,
online, 42, 44
Testosterone: "Muscle
with Attitude" Web
site, 74
The Body Web site,
250, 253
therapeutic interactions
of drugs or herbs, 230
therapies
alternative
medicine, 195
acupuncture, 197
Ayurveda, 197
Chinese, 197
chiropractic, 197
choosing, 199
Feldenkrais
Method, 198
macrobiotic
diets, 198
massage, 198-199
placebo effect, 200
scams, 201
mental health, 218
therapists, online, mental
health, 218-220
thigh muscles, exercising,
44, 180, 207
Thrive Online Web
site, 83

Thrive Web site, 242
Tile.net Web site, 23-24
time management,
  scheduling aerobic
  exercises, 56-57
timeliness (PILOT
  method), 35
tools
  online, personal fitness
    programs, 50-51
  research on Internet, 8
Topica Web site, 23
TOPS (Take Off Pounds
  Sensibly)
  Web site, 146
Total Fitness Guide Web
  site, 84
tracking progress with
  fitness programs, 49-51
trade publications, 21
traditional recipes, Web
  site, 179
trainers, personal
  advantages and
    disadvantages, 78
  certification, 79
  education, 79
  experience, 80
  fees, 80
  individualization, 80
  liability insurance, 80
  personality, 81
  policies, 80
  professionalism, 80
  qualifications, 79
  via email, 82-83
traveling
  exercising
    hotels with gyms,
      118-119
    resorts or spas,
      117-118
    vacations, 115-116

suitcases, lifting
  properly, 119
treadmills, online
  shopping, 106
treatments
  cancer, alternative,
    257-258
  HIV/AIDS, 249-250
  menopause, 240
    alternative, 241-243
    conventional, 241
  mental health, 218
triceps, exercising, 69
Tufts Nutrition Navigator
  Web site, 132-133
Turnstep.com
  Web site, 63
Twelve Reasons Every
  Adult Should Do
  Strength Exercise
  Web site, 66

U

unfiltered information on
  Internet, 8
University of California
  (Berkeley) Web site, 16
unmoderated
  bulletin boards, 24
  mailing lists, 23
  newsgroups, 24
US Swing Dance Server
  (The) Web site, 98
U.S. Department of
  Health and Human
  Services Web site, 201
U.S. Food and Drug
  Administration Web
  site, 141
U.S. National Library of
  Medicine (The) Web
  site, 188

V

vacations, exercising,
  113-116
vegetables
  broth, 176
  recommended
    servings, 175
vegetarians
  Fatfree: The Low Fat
    Vegetarian Recipe
    Archive Web site, 127
  meat, beans
    substituting, 126
Veggies Unite! Web
  site, 133
VegSource Web site, 178
Verified Internet
  Pharmacy Practice Sites
  (VIPPS seal), 227
Video Fitness Web
  site, 108
videos
  aerobics, 63
  exercise, 108
VIPPS (Verified Internet
  Pharmacy Practice Sites)
  seal, 227
Virtual Medical Center,
  Mediconsult.com Web
  site, 194
vitamins, 128
Vitamins Network Web
  site, 128
Voight, Karen, 83

W

walking, 59
Walking Club Web
  site, 59
Walking Connection
  Web site, 59

Walking Magazine Web site, 20
  best treadmill workouts, 62
Web directories, 16-17
Web pages, bookmarking, 19
Web sites. *See also* Internet
  24-Hour Fitness, 48
  About.com, 21
  ACE (American Council on Exercise), 84
  Active Videos, 108-109
  ActiveLog, 50
  ADA (American Dietetic Association), 129
  adam.com, 235
  Aerobics FAQ, 54
  AFAA (The Aerobics and Fitness Association of America), kickboxing, 63
  AIDS Health Fraud Task Force (Florida), 251
  AiKiWeb, 91
  AllHerb.com, 230-231
  AltaVista, 15, 18
  Alternative Health News Online, 203
  Alternative Medicine Online, 197
  AMA (American Medical Association), 43
  Amazon.com, 108
  America by Bicycle, 115

American Bodybuilding, 73
American Cancer Society (ACS), 256, 261
  Web sites warning, 258
American Chiropractic Association, 198
American Council on Exercise, 21, 58
American Heart Association, 141
American Institute for Cancer Research, 21
American Medical Association strength training, 71
AMTA (American Massage Therapy Association Message Therapy Journal, 198-199
Any Swing Goes, 98
APA (American Psychological Association) Web site, 218
Appalachian Long Distance Hikers Association (The), 95
Ask Dr. Weil, 202
Association of Cancer Online Resources Inc. (ACOR), 260
associations, 21
Avert, 248
Ayurvedic Institute (The), 197
BackWoods Grocery, 96
BallroomDancers.com, 99-100

Band-Aides and Blackboards, 209
Benny Goodsport, 101-102
Better Health, 260
Bicycling Magazine, 61
Bill Pearl, 73
Blonz Guide to Nutrition, Food & Health Resources, 134
Body Caliper, 109
Body Positive, 171-172
Bodybuilding Jargon, 73
BodyPump, 63
bookmarking, 19
Books-for-Cooks, 179
Brick Bodies, 48-49
British Medical Journal (The), 186
Brown brothers (Ken and Ron), 156
browsing, 16
"Buy Me" sites, 188
California Medical Association, 193
Calorie Control Council, 137, 143
CampUSA, 96
CancerGuide, 257, 260-261
CancerNet, 261
CanSearch, 263
CataList, 23
CDC (Centers for Disease Control and Prevention), 247
Center for Alternative Medicine Research (UT-CAM), 257
Center for Food Safety and Applied Nutrition, 141

Center for Science in the Public Interest, 38

Childbirth.org, 212

children's health, 209-212

Club Med, 116

Collage Video, 63, 108

Complete Guide to Strength Training (The), 70

Comprehensive Cancer Center, 259

Condomania, 248

Confessions of an Online Drug User, 227

conwebs, 184

Cook's Thesaurus, 174

CookeryBooks, 179

Cool Running, 60

Cory Everson's Guide to Working Out, 52

Country Walkers, 115

Critical Path Aids Project, 253

CrossTrak, 49

CSPI (Center for Science in the Public Interest), 133

CVS.com, 227-229

Cyber Cyclery, 62

CyberDiet, 124, 142

CyberDiet Buddies Forum, 148

CyberPump, 74

Dakota Fit Software, 49

Dearest, 243

Death and Dying, 217

DejaNews, 24

delusions about Internet, 217

Depression, 216

Diet Buddy, 150-151

Dietfraud, 156

Direct Information on Research and Treatment (DIRT), 252

DIRT (Direct Information on Research and Treatment), 252

Discovery Health, 193, 235, 244

Doctor's Guide to Menopause, 245

DogPile, 18

Dr. C. Everett Koop, MD, 8

Dr. Grohol's Mental Health Page, 221

Dr. Paula, 207

drkoop.com. 20
  aerobics, 63
  personal drugstore, 234

Drug Emporium, 227

DrugDigest.org, 234

Drugstore.com, 227

East Coast Swing, 99

Eating Disorders Awareness and Prevention, Inc., 169

Epicurious, 174

ethnic recipes, 179

evaluating, PILOT method, 30-36

exaggerated claims, 29

Excite, 15, 18

ExRx Online, 72

Facts About Weight Loss Products and Programs, 155

Familymeds.com, 227

FAQs (Frequently Asked Questions), 21

Fat City, weight-loss gimmicks, how to report, 156

Fatfree: The Low Fat Vegetarian Recipe Archive, 127

FDA, Guide to Choosing Medical Treatments, 200

fees charged, 31

Feldenkrais Guild of North America, 198

Fit @ Home, 105-106

Fit and Trim Support Group, 147

Fit for Business, 119

fitness activity, 21

Fitness Files, 46

Fitness Link, Find a Friend for Weight Loss Support, 150

Fitness Motivation, 66

Fitness Online, 71

Fitness Partner Connection Jumpsite, 10, 58
  Activity Calorie Calculator, 55
  cardiovascular machine workouts, 62

Fitness Products Council, 105

Fitness Registry, 107

Fitness Resource, 51

FitnessLink, 52, 105, 111, 129, 140, 155
  certification organizations, 79

mind/body
  exercising, 87
  Target Heart Rate
    Calculator, 57
  weight-loss books,
    evaluating, 159-160
FNIC (Food and
  Nutrition Information
  Center), 128
Fogdog, 106
Food Finder, 138
Food Guide
  Pyramid, 130
  A Guide to Daily
    Food Choices, 136
Forum One, 24, 148
FTC, Tips for Buying
  Exercise Equipment,
  104-105
Georgia State
  University, strength
  training, 71
Girl Power's Body
  Wise, 209-210
Global Health &
  Fitness, 72
Gold's Gym, 48
Goldenjane, 92
GORP (The Great
  Outdoor Recreation
  Pages), 94
GoTo, 18
Great Outdoors, 95
Hardin Meta Directory
  of Internet Health
  Sources, 193
Headworks, 218
Health and Fitness
  Network, 84
Health Central, 11
HealthAtoZ, 10
HealthBoards.com, 189

HealthCentral, 20, 36,
  187, 193, 217
HealthClubs.com, 48
Healthfinder, 37, 193
Healthscout, 28,
  203, 232
HealthWeb, 194, 202
HealthWeb AIDS, 254
Healthwell.com, 231
HealthWorld Online,
  Chinese
  medicine, 197
Healthy Fridge, 210
Healthy Refrigerator,
  174-175
Healthy Weight
  Network, 160, 171
HealthyKids.com, 211
Herb Research
  Foundation
  (The), 230
Herbal Minefield
  (The), 232
HerbMed, 231
HIV and
  Hepatitis.com, 253
HIV InSite, 253
HIV/AIDS Information
  Center, 251
HIV/AIDS Testing, 249
HIV/AIDS Treatment
  Information
  Service, 250
Hot Flash, 243
HotBot, 15, 18
How to Increase the
  Amount of Fiber in
  your Diet, 125
IDEA, The Health and
  Fitness Source, 78
IMBA (International
  Mountain Biking
  Association), 95

institutions, 21
InteliHealth, 194
International Food
  Information Council,
  38, 188
International
  Sivananda Yoga
  Vedanta Centers, 89
Internet FAQ
  Consortium, 21
Internet Squash
  Federation, 60
IRC (Internet Relay
  Chat), 25
iVillage allHealth, 235
JAMA (Journal of the
  American Medical
  Association), 186
JanaTrains, 57
Jazzercise, 63
Jean-Paul Fitness
  Specialists, 72
Jenny Craig, 142
Joan Price, 45, 119
John Lee, M.D., 242
Judo, 92
Jujutsu, 92
jump sites, 19
Kick It, 99
kidsDoctor, 206
KidsHealth.org,
  209-211
KidSource, 206
L.L. Bean's Park
  Search, 94
Leya Aum, 219
Life Form, 50
Lindy Hop, 98
Liszt, 23-25
look of, 34
Looksmart, 17-18

Losing Weight—An Ill-Fated New Year's Resolution, 167

Low-Fat Vegetarian Recipe Archive, 178

Macrobiotics Online, 198

magazines, 21

Martial Arts Resource Page, 91

Mayo Clinic, 194

Mayo Clinic Health Oasis Nutrition Center, 128, 132

MD Consult, 188

Meals For You, 180

MediConsult, 194

Mediconsult.com, 11

Medscape, 194

Menopause Guidebook, 244

Menopause mailing list, 243

Menopause Resource Guide, 245

menopause.org, 242

Mental Health, 222

Mental Health at iVillage, 221

Mental Health Net, 216, 222

Mental Health Resources About.Com, 222

Mental Health Resources Guide at About.com, 220

Menopause FAQs, 244

Metanoia, 219

metasearch, 17-18

metasites, health/ medical, 193-194

Mind Tools: Sport Psychology, 92

Montana, 106

Mrznet, 97

Muscle & Fitness Magazine Online, 74

Mylifepath.com, 124

Myria, 208

National Association of Boards of Pharmacy, 227

National Cancer Institute (NCI), 261

National Food Safety Database, 177

National Institute of Aging, 245

National Pasta Association, 177

National Women's Health Information Center, 245

NCAM (National Center for Complementary and Alternative Medicine), 202

NetGrocer, 177

NetPsychology, 223

NetPsychology.com, 220

Netsweat, 107

New England Journal of Medicine (The), 167, 186-187

New York Online Access to Health (NOAH), 262

NewRunner.com, 60

news sites, 19-20

NIH (National Institutes of Health), 221

NNF (Nutrition News Focus), 132

NOAH (New York Online Access to Health) Web site, 202

NordiCaLite, 163

North American Menopause Society, 241 linking, 245

Nourish Net Club, 143

OA (Overeaters Anonymous), 146

OARS (Outdoor Adventure River Specialists), 116

OncoLink, 259, 262

ONElist, 23

OnHealth, 20, 194

Online Stretches, 88

Ornish, 126

Outdoor Explorer, 94

Outward Bound, 116

ParentsPlace, 208

ParentsPlace.com, 211

Periodization of Strength, 74

personal, 22

Phys.com, 88

PHYS: Snack Bandit, 95

Pilates-Studio, 90

PlanetRx, 227

Polar, 109

Pregnancy at About.com, 212

Pregnancy Today, 208, 212

Pro Track 99, 49

Psych Central, 221

Public Eye (The), 110

Publicly Accessible Mailing Lists, 23

quack weight-loss sites
   identifying, 160
Quackwatch, 37, 105
   cancer quack
      treatments, 257
   cellulite
      removal, 161
   weight-loss
      gimmicks, 156
Quackwatch.com, 232
Racewalk, 59
Radiance, 168, 170
Randolfi, 38
recipes, 180
   sharing, 178
Recreation at
   About.com, 95
reliability, 29
Reuters Health
   eLine, 20
Richard Simmons,
   118, 149
Rob Wood's Fitness
   Testing, 43
Rollerblade.com, 59-60
Rx.com, 227
SaferSex.org, 248
Samaritans (The), 216
SavoyStyle Swing
   Dance Shop, 98
SavvySearch, 18
scams, strength
   training, 72
Search Engine
   Showdown, 14
Self-Care Advisor:
   Menopause, 240
Shape Up America,
   101, 144
Shape Up America
   Fitness Club
   Assessment, 43

Share the Hope &
   Humor, 259
Sierra Club, 96
Skating.com, 59
Ski Travel Online, 116
SkiCentral, 96
Snack Bandit, 95
Snap, 17-18
SOAR (Searchable
   Online Archive of
   Recipes), 178, 180
Something Fishy Web
   site on Eating
   Disorders (The), 169
Southern Medical
   Journal, 217
Spa Magazine, 118
Spa-Finder, 117
Spinning, 63
Sports Parents, 101
StarChefs, 179
storefront, 22
StorkSite, 212
Stott Conditioning, 90
STOTT Pilates Studios
   & International
   Certification
   Center, 90
Strength Training and
   Women, 67
strength-assessment
   test, 70
Strong Women, 69
Strong, Stretched &
   Centered Mind-Body
   Fitness Training
   Institute, 86
Suicide: Read This
   First, 216
Swim 2000, 61
SwimInfo, 61
Switcheroo, 174
Tai Chi, 92

Tanita, 109
TennisLinks.com, 60
Testosterone: "Muscle
   with Attitude," 74
The Body, 250, 253
Thrive, 242
Thrive Online, 83
Tile.net, 23-24
Topica, 23
TOPS (Take Off Pounds
   Sensibly), 146
Total Fitness Guide, 84
trade publications, 21
traditional recipes, 179
Tufts Nutrition
   Navigator, 132-133
Turnstep.com, 63
Twelve Reasons Every
   Adult Should Do
   Strength Exercise, 66
types of, 19
University of
   California
   (Berkeley), 16
US Swing Dance Server
   (The), 98
U.S. Department of
   Health and Human
   Services, 201
U.S. Food and Drug
   Administration, 141
U.S. National Library
   of Medicine
   (The), 188
Veggies Unite!, 133
VegSource, 178
Video Fitness, 108
Vitamins Network, 128
Walking Club, 59
Walking
   Connection, 59
Walking Magazine, 20
   best treadmill
      workouts, 62

WebMD, 199, 201
Wegmans Food
  Stores, 176
weight loss, 142-144
  evaluating with
    PILOT method, 141
Weight Watchers,
  145, 155
Weight-control
  Information
  Network, 140
Weight.com,
  weight-loss
  gimmicks, 155
Weighty Matters, 74
WellnessWeb, 202
West Coast Swing, 99
Women's Quest Fitness
  Camps, 116
Workoutlog.com, 51
Worldwide Outdoor
  Adventures, 116
WWW Martial Arts
  Resource Page, 91
Yahoo!, 17-18,
  107, 110
    Mental Wellness
      Club, 221
    Yoga Site, 89
YOGAaahhh, 89
Zoftig Zone, 171
WebMD Web site,
  199, 201
Wegmans Food Stores
  Web site, 176
weight
  exercise, calories
    used, 9
  genetic factors,
    166-167
  healthy lifestyles,
    167-169
  loss/control, 55

self-acceptance,
  166, 169-172
set point, 165-166
weight loss, 135
  adults, statistics, 168
  BMI (Body Mass
    Index), 140
  books, 158
    evaluating, 159-160
  calories, 136-137, 143
  children, statistics, 169
  exercising, 138-139
  expectations
    (unrealistic), 139
  gimmicks
    Brown brothers,
      156, 158
    how to report, Fat
      City Web site, 156
    Quackwatch Web
      site, 156
    Weight.com Web
      site, 155
  healthy lifestyles,
    167-169
  junk food, 137-138
  maintenance
    programs,
    choosing, 141
  programs
    choosing, 140-141
    commercial, 142
    maintenance,
    choosing, 141
  quack weight-loss sites,
    identifying, 160
  researching, 140-141
  scams
    burns fat, 161
    buzzwords, 162
    cellulite
      removal, 161
    junk mail, 159

no diets or
  exercise, 162
recognizing,
  154-158, 160-162
testing, 163-164
support groups
  bulletin boards,
    148-149
  chat rooms, 148
  commercial, 145-146
  email pen pals, 150
  mailing lists, 147
  newsgroups, 147
  OA (Overeaters
    Anonymous) Web
    site, 146
  online, 147-150
  TOPS (Take Off
    Pounds Sensibly)
    Web site, 146
  Weight Watchers
    Web site, 145
Web sites, 142-144
  evaluating with
    PILOT method, 141
Weight-control
  Information Network
  Web site, 140
weight training, strength
  training, 65
  advantages of, 66
  anxiety reducer, 66
  basics, 67
  bodybuilding, 73
  muscles, 67
  results, 70
  scams, Web sites, 72
  scheduling
    exercises, 68
  sets, 68
  strength-assessment
    test, 70
  stress reducer, 66

weights, 69
for women, 67
Weight Watchers Web
site, 145, 155
Weight-control
Information Network
Web site, 140
Weight.com Web site,
weight-loss
gimmicks, 155
weights, strength
training, 68-69
Weights Web site,
mailing list, 74
Weighty Matters
Web site, 74
Weil, Andrew, 202
WellnessWeb
Web site, 202
Wernick, Sarah, 69
Wescott, Wayne L., 66
West Coast Swing
Web site, 99
Winfrey, Oprah, 158
Wistie, Shelly, 150
women
caloric needs,
calculating, 124
HRT (hormone
replacement
therapy), 241
menopause, 245
alternative
treatment, 241-243
conventional
treatment, 241
support groups, 243
symptoms, 239-240
treatment, 240-243
National Institute of
Aging, 245

North American
Menopause
Society, 244
perimenopause, 240
phytoestrogens, 244
strength training, 67
weight loss,
statistics, 168
Women's Quest Fitness
Camps Web site, 116
words, buzzwords for diet
scams, 162
Workoutlog.com Web
site, 51
World Squash
Federation, 60
World Wide Web. *See*
WWW
Worldwide Outdoor
Adventures Web
site, 116
WWW (World Wide
Web), 8. *See also*
Internet; Web sites
hyperlinks, 9

X-Z

Yahoo! Web site, 17-18,
107, 110
Mental Wellness
Club, 221
yoga, mind/body
exercising, 88-89
Yoga Site Web site, 89
YOGAaahhh Web site, 89

Zoftig Zone Web site, 171

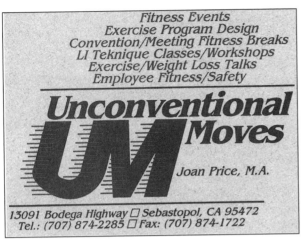
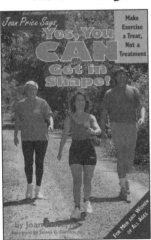
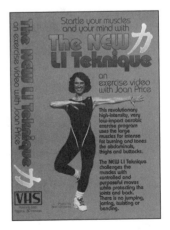

Just Eat It! Don't Eat It! Eat it! Don't Eat It.

Just Do It! Don't Do It! Do It. Don't Do It.

Visit FitnessLink at
`http://www.`
`fitnesslink.com`

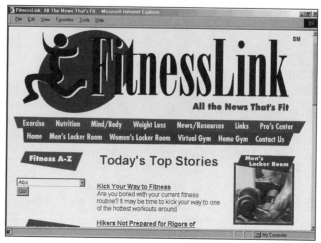

It's easy to be confused about what's best for your body when the mainstream media reports alarming news that actually conflicts with yesterday's alarming news. For the truth about losing weight, burning fat, working out, bulking up, staying motivated, taking herbs and vitamins, and feeling happy with yourself, turn to FitnessLink. No fluff. No nonsense. We go beyond the sound bites and tell it like it is, revealing the real-life experiences of professional athletes, fitness instructors, sports trainers, physicians, and nutritionists as well as everyday people who work hard and play hard. FitnessLink strives to help people make informed decisions about their health and the health of their families and ultimately to spark inspiration and happiness.

And from FitnessLink, you can link to every hot link in this book.

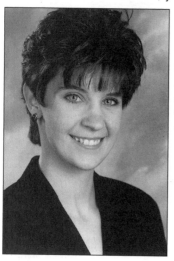

FitnessLink is the realization of a dream: my dream to help people get fit and stay there, to help them unlock their abilities, both mental and physical, through fitness. By merging my online publishing skills with my love of fitness, I use the Internet to promote fitness education to millions of people around the world! And the feedback I've received confirms that people are finding the knowledge and support they need through FitnessLink.